# 100 Questions & Answers About Kidney Cancer

## SECOND EDITION

### Steven C. Campbell, MD, PhD
*Cleveland Clinic/
Glickman Urological & Kidney Institute
Cleveland, OH*

### Brian I. Rini, MD, FACP
*Cleveland Clinic/
Glickman Urological & Kidney Institute
Cleveland, OH*

### Robert G. Uzzo, MD, FACS
*Division of Urologic Oncology
Fox Chase Cancer Center
Temple University School of Medicine
Philadelphia, PA*

### Brian R. Lane, MD, PhD
*Chief of Urology at Spectrum Health Regional Cancer Center
Michigan State University College of Human Medicine
Grand Rapids, MI*

### Stephanie Chisolm, PhD
*Patient Educator*

JONES & BARTLETT
LEARNING

*World Headquarters*
Jones & Bartlett Learning
5 Wall Street
Burlington, MA 01803
978-443-5000
info@jblearning.com
www.jblearning.com

Jones & Bartlett Learning books and products are available through most bookstores and online booksellers. To contact Jones & Bartlett Learning directly, call 800-832-0034, fax 978-443-8000, or visit our website, www.jblearning.com.

Substantial discounts on bulk quantities of Jones & Bartlett Learning publications are available to corporations, professional associations, and other qualified organizations. For details and specific discount information, contact the special sales department at Jones & Bartlett Learning via the above contact information or send an email to specialsales@jblearning.com.

The content, statements, views, and opinions herein are the sole expression of the respective authors and not that of Jones & Bartlett Learning, LLC. Reference herein to any specific commercial product, process, or service by trade name, trademark, manufacturer, or otherwise does not constitute or imply its endorsement or recommendation by Jones & Bartlett Learning, LLC and such reference shall not be used for advertising or product endorsement purposes. All trademarks displayed are the trademarks of the parties noted herein. *100 Questions & Answers About Kidney Cancer, Second Edition* is an independent publication and has not been authorized, sponsored, or otherwise approved by the owners of the trademarks or service marks referenced in this product.

There may be images in this book that feature models; these models do not necessarily endorse, represent, or participate in the activities represented in the images. Any screenshots in this product are for educational and instructive purposes only. Any individuals and scenarios featured in the case studies throughout this product may be real or fictitious, but are used for instructional purposes only.

The authors, editor, and publisher have made every effort to provide accurate information. However, they are not responsible for errors, omissions, or for any outcomes related to the use of the contents of this book and take no responsibility for the use of the products and procedures described. Treatments and side effects described in this book may not be applicable to all people; likewise, some people may require a dose or experience a side effect that is not described herein. Drugs and medical devices are discussed that may have limited availability controlled by the Food and Drug Administration (FDA) for use only in a research study or clinical trial. Research, clinical practice, and government regulations often change the accepted standard in this field. When consideration is being given to use of any drug in the clinical setting, the health care provider or reader is responsible for determining FDA status of the drug, reading the package insert, and reviewing prescribing information for the most up-to-date recommendations on dose, precautions, and contraindications, and determining the appropriate usage for the product. This is especially important in the case of drugs that are new or seldom used.

**Production Credits**

VP, Executive Publisher: David D. Cella
Executive Acquisitions Editor: Nancy Anastasi Duffy
Editorial Assistant: Jade Freeman
Production Assistant: Alex Schab
Digital Marketing Manager: Jennifer Sharp
Manufacturing and Inventory Control Supervisor: Amy Bacus
Composition: Miranda Design Studio, Inc.
Cover Design: Kristin E. Parker
Rights and Media Research Coordinator: Ashley Dos Santos
Cover Image: Top Left: © Yuri Arcurs/ShutterStock, Inc.
Top Right: © Ryan McVay/Photodisc/Getty Images
Bottom: © Alexander Raths/ShutterStock, Inc.
Printing and Binding: Edwards Brothers Malloy
Cover Printing: Edwards Brothers Malloy

**Library of Congress Cataloging-in-Publication Data**
Campbell, Steven C., 1959-
  100 questions and answers about kidney cancer / Steven C. Campbell, Brian I. Rini, Robert G. Uzzo. — Second edition.
    pages cm
  title: Hundred and one questions and answers about kidney cancer
  title: Hundred one questions and answers about kidney cancer
  ISBN 978-1-284-03857-6
1. Kidneys—Cancer—Miscellanea. 2. Kidneys—Cancer—Popular works. I. Rini, Brian I. II. Uzzo, Robert G. III. Title.
IV. Title: Hundred and one questions and answers about kidney cancer. V. Title: Hundred one questions and answers about kidney cancer.
  RC280.K5C34 2014
  616.99'461—dc23

6048

Printed in the United States of America
19 18 17 16 15      10 9 8 7 6 5 4 3 2 1

# CONTENTS

# *Introduction*

A diagnosis of cancer is one of the most stressful of life's occurrences for a variety of reasons—fear of pain, fear of side effects of treatment, and fear of death. But there is another thing that happens that is almost as distressing—fear of the unknown. For most patients and their families, encountering the medical system in its full glory is a very confusing and disorienting experience. Often, the questions they have are very simple: what is this cancer and why me? But, given the time constraints of modern medical practice, even the most dedicated of physicians will need to focus primarily on management issues—what treatments should be considered and what are their advantages and disadvantages? Many patients have a hard time concentrating during these counseling sessions—they are often too preoccupied with fundamental concerns (how long do I have to live?), and they do not process information well. Many patients feel a profound sense of loss of control, and this is one of the most distressing aspects of the whole experience.

For patients with kidney cancer, which can be a lethal malignancy, all of these issues are magnified.

So what can we do about this? Where can a patient turn to learn more about kidney cancer?

The Internet is always a good place to start—it's free, easy to access, and represents a wealth of information. However, therein lies the problem—it provides too much information, most of which does not apply to the patient's situation. Even more importantly, there are too many infomercials. More than 80% of the medical-related information on the Internet has a hidden agenda. In many cases, it is not so hidden if you know the field. Additionally, some of the information is just not very accurate. Some of it is better classified as myth, rumor, or wild exaggeration. It is easy to get misled.

The purpose of this book is to provide the essential information about kidney cancer that will bring you "up to speed" about your diagnosis. Its design—simple questions and answers—will parallel your concerns and empower you with information. It is not meant to be read from cover to cover, although this is allowed if you so desire. Rather, it is probably better to start with what-ever you find most interesting or distressing about your particular situation, and then move forward from there.

The first section covers the basics, such as what kidney cancer is, what the kidneys are, and what they do. The causes and risk factors for developing kidney cancer are then addressed, followed by a review of the common symptoms of kidney cancer and an overview of how patients are evaluated and staged. The treatments of kidney cancer are then discussed, broken down by the stage of the cancer: localized (still confined to the kid-neys), locally advanced (breaking out of the kidney or into the lymph nodes), or metastatic (spread to other parts of the body). In the process, we review all of the basic treatment options for kidney cancer, ranging from watch and wait, surgical removal or ablation, chemo-therapy, immunotherapy, and the targeted molecular treatments that have revolutionized the field. We have tried to do all of this in layman's terms. Our goal is to explain it to you clearly as if we were sitting right in front of you.

If our excitement about the field of kidney cancer shines through, that is not a mistake. Kidney cancer has become arguably the most interesting and challenging of all of the cancers in modern oncology. Great research, surgical, and medical advances have occurred recently that allow us to treat our patients more effectively and, in general, with less severe side effects. But with this has come increased complexity. Each patient must now consider a variety of options and weigh out what is best for their particular situation. Hopefully, this book will help you as you work through this process.

We would like to thank Stephanie Chisolm, PhD, for her great assistance with this project, particularly with helping us avoid too much medical lingo and making the text easy to read and understand. This book would not have come together without Stephanie's help. Great gratitude is also due to the caregivers and patients who provided commentary about many of the topics in this book—this has helped to bring a real life perspective to these issues.

We would also like to thank our mentors in the field of urologic oncology for their example and dedication, including Andrew Novick, Ron Bukowski, Eric Klein, Robert Flanigan, Jim Finke, and Paul Russo. Finally, our gratitude to our families for their support and encouragement cannot be adequately expressed, certainly not in the limited space available here.

**Steven C. Campbell, MD, PhD**
**Brian I. Rini, MD, FACP**
**Robert G. Uzzo, MD, FACS**
**Brian R. Lane, MD, PhD**

# PART ONE

# *The Basics*

What is kidney cancer?

Where are the kidneys located in the body?

What do the kidneys normally do?

*More*[*]...

## Cancer

An uncontrolled growth of cells.

## Kidney

Either of the two organs in the lumbar region that filter the blood, excreting the end-products of body metabolism in the form of urine, and regulating the concentrations of hydrogen, sodium, potassium, phosphate, and other ions in the extracellular fluid.

## Abdomen

The cavity of the body containing the stomach, intestines, liver, and spleen. The kidneys are located behind this cavity.

## Carcinogen

Any substance or agent that tends to produce a cancer.

## Urine

Liquid waste product filtered from the blood by the kidneys, stored in the bladder, and expelled from the body through the urethra by the act of urinating (voiding). About 96% of urine is water, with the remaining 4% being comprised of waste products.

## Renal cell carcinoma (RCC)

Cancer of the kidney.

# 1. What is kidney cancer?

Kidney cancer is **cancer** that begins in the **kidneys**, which are organs that lie in the back of the **abdomen**, behind the bowels. The kidneys are the main filters of the body. They filter out waste products and **carcinogens** (cancer-causing substances), transferring them from the bloodstream into the **urine**. These undesirable substances can then be eliminated from the body. Another common name for kidney cancer is **renal cell carcinoma (RCC)**. **Renal** refers to the kidney, a **cell** is the smallest unit of our living bodies, and **carcinoma** is another name for cancer.

Cancer is an uncontrolled growth of cells that eventually become large enough to make a **tumor**. Normal cells divide only when needed to replace other cells that are dying and this process is very tightly regulated. Cancer cells have **mutations** that allow them to divide out of control; the body is often unable to stop this process. The tumor cells also become resistant to the natural cycle of growth and cell death (also known as **apoptosis**), and they just keep growing. Cancer cells also **secrete** certain **proteins (proteases)** that can digest the surrounding tissue, allowing the cells to invade adjacent areas. The tumor cells can then spread to other parts of the body; this is known as **metastasis**. The tumor cells can also stimulate new blood vessels to grow toward them to provide nutrients and oxygen for continued growth. This is known as **angiogenesis**—without angiogenesis the tumor cells would starve or remain dormant (inactive). A cancer cell must be able to do most or all of these things to metastasize, cause pain, or kill a patient. Unfortunately, some kidney cancers have this potential. Tumors that have this potential are called **malignant**. Tumors that cannot invade locally or metastasize are

**benign**—these tumors can grow, but rarely cause trouble and can often be left untreated.

Kidney cancer has always been relatively unresponsive to **chemotherapy**, which is somewhat unique in the cancer world. The main hope for most kidney cancer patients is that the cancer can be removed surgically—kidney cancer is still primarily a surgical disease. However, thanks to the work of dedicated researchers and clinicians, better treatments are now available for all stages of kidney cancer, even for patients with more advanced disease that cannot be removed surgically. New treatments that block the blood vessels supplying tumors with nutrients and oxygen can starve the tumor and slow or reverse its growth. These treatments, known as **anti-angiogenic treatments**, have created great excitement for the treatment of patients with kidney cancer and have moved kidney cancer to the forefront of modern **oncology**.

## 2. Where are the kidneys located in the body?

Most people have two kidneys and the usual location is in the back of the abdomen, behind the **bowels**. Typically, there is one kidney on each side of the body. The kidneys lie near the top of the abdomen, just inside the muscles that surround the abdomen (**Figure 1**). The bowels, liver, pancreas, and other organs sit in front of the kidneys within a lining called the **peritoneum**. The kidneys are located in the area known as the **flank** or the **retroperitoneum**, literally meaning "behind the peritoneum."

Under normal conditions the kidneys cannot be **palpated** or felt by external examination, because they are shielded

**Renal**
Relating to the kidney.

**Cell**
The smallest unit of life that is classified as a living thing. Each cell contains all of the basic structural and functional components of living organisms, also known as the building blocks of life.

**Carcinoma**
An invasive malignant tumor derived from epithelial tissue that tends to metastasize to other areas of the body.

**Tumor**
An abnormal growth of tissue, which can be benign or malignant. Similar to the term neoplasm, but should be distinguished from the term cancer, which implies at least some malignant potential.

**Mutations**
Changes in chromosomes or genes that cause proteins to function abnormally and begin a "cancerous process." Mutations can be caused by the effects of chemicals, radiation, or even ordinary heat on DNA.

THE BASICS

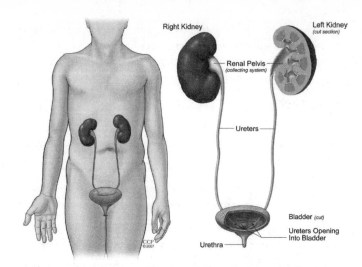

**Figure 1a** The kidneys are found just below the ribcage behind the contents of the abdomen. The kidneys filter the blood and make urine which drains through the ureters and into the bladder.

Reprinted with permission, Cleveland Clinic Center for Medical Art & Photography. © 2007–2014. All Rights Reserved.

by the bowels and other organs. The lower part of the rib cage is also in the way. Because the kidneys are hidden or **"sequestered"** in the back of the abdomen, many patients with kidney cancer can have a fairly large tumor without knowing about it. These tumors often cannot be felt and many patients do not have symptoms until the cancer spills blood into the urine, compresses a nerve leading to pain, or creates symptoms in some other way. For this reason, the majority of patients with kidney cancer currently present without symptoms, or incidentally.

## 3. What do the kidneys normally do?

The kidneys are the main filters of the body. They remove waste products and carcinogens (cancer-causing substances), transferring them from the bloodstream into the urine. These undesirable substances can then be eliminated from the body. Each kidney has one or

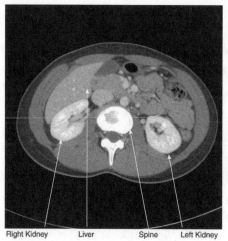

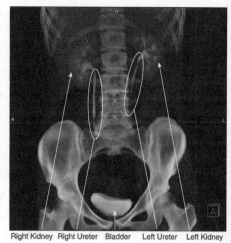

Right Kidney    Liver    Spine    Left Kidney

Right Kidney    Right Ureter    Bladder    Left Ureter    Left Kidney

**Figure 1b**  Normal appearance of the kidneys on computed tomography (CT) scan. This image shows one section of the body as if the patient were sliced across the abdomen while laying face-up (axial or transverse slice). The image was obtained shortly after intravenous (I.V.) contrast has been given, in order to demonstrate the uptake of dye within the filtering portion of the kidneys.

**Figure 1c**  A reconstruction of several axial CT images can show the kidneys as they would appear if you were looking directly into a person standing in front of you (coronal view). This radiograph is a delayed image that depicts contrast within the collection and drainage system of the kidney.

more **arteries** to supply blood and one or more **veins** that drain the blood back toward the heart. The blood flow through the kidney is tremendous, almost equal to that of the brain. This filtering function is so important to our health and well being that one-quarter of all the blood that is pumped out of the heart goes into the kidneys. When the kidneys are not working, waste products build up in the bloodstream and slow our mental activity and make us feel sick. Prolonged shut down of the kidneys can cause death.

Each kidney has about a million microscopic filters called **glomeruli**. As the blood passes through the glomeruli, waste products and other undesirable substances are removed and passed into the urine. In addition, the

**Angiogenesis**

The formation of new blood vessels, especially blood vessels that supply oxygen and nutrients to cancerous tissues.

**Malignant**

The term literally means growing worse and resisting treatment. It is used as a synonym for cancerous and connotes a harmful condition that generally is life threatening.

**Benign**

Of no danger to health; not recurrent or progressive; not malignant: a benign tumor.

**Chemotherapy**

The treatment of cancer using specific chemical agents or drugs that are selectively destructive to malignant cells and tissues.

**Anti-angiogenic treatment**

Medication that prevents cancer growth by limiting the growth of new blood vessels that provide nutrients for cancer expansion.

**Oncology**

The branch of medicine that deals with the diagnosis and treatment of cancer.

**Bowels**

The intestines.

**Peritoneum**

The serous membrane lining the walls of the abdominal and pelvic cavities and investing the contained viscera , the two layers enclosing a potential space, the peritoneal cavity.

salt and acid/base balance of the blood is adjusted in a very precise manner that is controlled by the glomeruli and tubules of the kidneys. **High blood pressure** and **diabetes** are two common diseases that can lead to gradual damage and loss of kidney function in part by damaging these delicate microscopic filters.

Patients with **kidney failure** must consider **dialysis** or kidney **transplantation**. The most common treatment for kidney failure is dialysis, whereby a patient is connected to a machine that filters the blood outside of the body. Each dialysis session takes about 3–4 hours and most patients are dialyzed 3 days each week. This treatment works well enough to keep the patient alive and functional, but is never as effective as the natural kidneys. The second option is kidney transplantation, where a kidney is obtained from a loved one or accident victim and surgically placed into the body. In order to maintain the kidney transplant, patients require **immunosuppressive medications** to allow their bodies to tolerate the new organ. Without these medications, the body's **immune system** would attack the transplanted kidney, a process also known as "**rejection**." With effective immunosuppression, the immune system is "tricked" into keeping the new kidney, but the patient is put at higher risk for infections because their immune system is weakened. Also, patients with a history of cancer are often required to wait at least a year or 2, and occasionally longer, to prove that they are cancer-free before they can receive a kidney transplant.

## 4. How is kidney function measured?

The standard measure of kidney function is the blood level of creatinine, also known as the **serum creatinine** level. **Creatinine** is a breakdown product of muscle that is released into the bloodstream when muscle cells die. Even in healthy people a small percentage of muscle cells die every day and these are replaced with new muscle cells. When cells die they release creatinine, so there is always some of this substance in the blood. If the kidneys are working normally, they filter creatinine out of the blood and eliminate it into the urine, driving down the blood creatinine levels. A low serum creatinine level indicates healthy kidneys. If the kidneys are not working well, the serum creatinine levels will rise. A normal serum creatinine level is about 1.0 mg/dl. An increase in serum creatinine level above 1.4 mg/dl indicates that the kidneys are beginning to malfunction, and when the serum creatinine level goes above 3.0 mg/dl, the level of concern becomes much greater. Older patients tend to have less muscle mass and lower serum creatinine values. In these patients, even small rises in the serum creatinine level can indicate loss of kidney function.

Because creatinine levels can vary according to gender, race, and body size, experts have developed formulas that better describe the level of kidney function. The **glomerular filtration rate**, or **GFR**, can be estimated based on serum creatinine or measured directly by specific testing that is more complex and costly than a simple blood test. A GFR value above 60 ml/min/1.73m$^2$ is considered normal and if measured directly can equal 100 or more. Kidney failure occurs only if GFR falls to below 15. Doctors and patients sometimes use the GFR value to give a picture of overall kidney function as a percentage of normal (100%). When the GFR falls to 50, the kidneys are working at about 50% of their normal function, but there remains a lot of reserve before dialysis may be necessary.

**Flank**

The side of a human, also known as the retroperitoneum. This is where the kidney can be asccessed during open or laparoscopic surgery, or by biopsy.

**Retroperitoneal**

The space between the peritoneum and the posterior abdominal wall that contains the kidneys, adrenal glands, pancreas, and part of the aorta and inferior vena cava.

**Palpate**

To examine by feeling and pressing with the palms of the hands and the fingers.

**Sequester**

To detach or separate abnormally a small portion from the whole.

**Arteries**

Blood vessels that carry blood to an organ, such as the kidney.

**Vein**

Blood vessel that carries blood away from an organ, such as the kidney.

THE BASICS

# *Key Term Definitions* (continued)

### Glomeruli

Glomeruli are knots of blood vessels in the kidney where the blood flows in, the urine is produced, and then the filtered blood flows out.

### High blood pressure

Elevation of the arterial blood pressure, also known as hypertension.

### Diabetes

A metabolic disorder in which excessive amounts of glucose (sugar) are found within the bloodstream. Generally refers to one of the two types of diabetes mellitus, insulin-dependent and non-insulin-dependent.

### Kidney failure

Inability of the kidneys to excrete waste, which results in a person's inability to maintain a balance of fluid and electrolytes, such as sodium and potassium.

### Immuno-suppressive medication

Drugs given to a transplant recipient to prevent his or her immune system from attacking the transplanted organ.

### Immune system

The body system that protects the organism by distinguishing foreign tissue and neutralizing potentially pathogenic organisms or substances. The immune system includes cells involved in the immune response, such as lymphocytes, and cell products such as lymphokines.

### Serum creatinine

The creatinine blood test measures the level of creatinine in the blood. This test is done to see how well your kidneys work.

### Creatinine

A breakdown product of muscle that is filtered by the kidney and measured in the blood or urine to provide an estimate of kidney function.

### Glomerular filtration rate (GFR)

A test to determine how well the kidneys are working. The estimate is based on the rate at which the kidneys filter the waste product creatinine from the bloodstream. According to the National Kidney Foundation, normal values range between 90 and 120 ml/min/1.73m$^2$. GFR values fall with age, so older people generally have lower values.

# PART TWO

# Causes and Risk Factors for Kidney Cancer

How common is kidney cancer?

Are there different types of kidney cancer?

What causes kidney cancer?

*More*...

## 5. How common is kidney cancer?

Kidney cancer is diagnosed in more than 64,000 patients each year in the United States, and each year about 13,000 patients will die of this cancer. It is estimated that 1 in every 10,000 people in this country will be diagnosed with kidney cancer each year. Kidney cancer is not one of the most common cancers such as prostate cancer, breast cancer, lung cancer, or colon cancer. And yet kidney cancer is not rare—overall it is the 9th or 10th most common cancer in the human body.

Kidney cancer is most often seen in people between the ages of 55 and 75, but can also occur in the young and the elderly. Sixty percent of the cases are in men and 40% are in women. Unfortunately, kidney cancer is on the rise—the rates of diagnosis have been going up about 3% each year for the past several years. The reasons for this are not entirely clear. Increased use of **CT scans** (also known as **CAT scans**) and **ultrasounds** to evaluate patients with stomach aches and other non-specific symptoms may be a contributing factor. These tests often reveal small, slow-growing tumors that might otherwise remain undiscovered. However, in addition to detecting more incidental cancers, we are also seeing more advanced and potentially **lethal** kidney cancers each year, and the reason for this more alarming finding is not known.

## 6. Are there different types of kidney cancer?

Over the past several years, doctors have learned that there are several different types of kidney cancer (**Table 1**). Each type has a distinctive appearance under the microscope and each is caused by distinct **genetic mutations**. To some

**CT scan (CAT scan)**

A "computerized tomography" (CT) or "computerized axial tomography" (CAT) scan uses a computer that takes data from several X-ray images of structures inside a human's or animal's body and converts them into pictures on a monitor.

**Ultrasound (US)**

An imaging modality that relies on sound waves that are transmitted through the skin, into the body, and detected by a transducer.

**Lethal**

Capable of causing death.

**Genetic mutation**

Change in the individual nucleotides of a gene that result in a change in the function or amount of that gene's protein product. Most nucleotide changes have no effect ("silent mutation"), but other mutations can have minor or major effects that can lead to disordered cell growth and cancer.

extent, each one has a typical pattern of clinical behavior, although there are many exceptions to these rules.

The most common type of kidney cancer is known as **clear cell renal cell carcinoma (RCC).** This represents about 75–80% of all kidney cancers. These tumors tend to be very **vascular** (having increased blood flow in and out), and on average they have a tendency to be more aggressive than the other common variants of kidney cancer. Most are caused by mutations of the **von Hippel-Lindau gene** on chromosome 3.

The next most common type of kidney cancer is known as **papillary RCC.** These represent about 10–15% of all kidney cancers. Most are caused by mutations or abnormalities of chromosomes 7 and 17. These tumors are usually not **hypervascular,** but they can be **multifocal**—many are associated with additional small tumors in the same kidney, known as **satellite lesions**. On average they tend to be less aggressive, but about 10% are atypical and can behave in a very aggressive manner.

**Clear cell renal cell carcinoma**

Most common type of kidney cancer, representing 70–80% of all cases of renal cell carcinoma, generally characterized by cells with clear cytoplasm. Genetic event responsible for this subtype is mutation or inactivation of the VHL gene on chromosome 3.

**Vascular**

Pertaining to, composed of, or provided with vessels or ducts that convey fluids, as blood or lymph.

**von Hippel-Lindau (VHL) gene**

The von Hippel–Lindau tumor suppressor also known as pVHL is a protein that in humans is encoded by the VHL gene.

**Papillary renal cell carcinoma**

The second most common subtype of kidney cancer, responsible for 10–15% of RCC. It is often multifocal with multiple lesions within one or both kidneys. Tends to display less aggressive clinical behavior.

**Table 1** Types of Kidney Cancer or Renal Cell Carcinoma (RCC)

| Type | Genetic Factors | Distinct Features | Behavior |
|------|-----------------|-------------------|----------|
| Clear cell RCC | Mutation of chromosome 3 | Hypervascular | Relatively aggressive in many patients |
| Papillary RCC | Abnormalities of chromosomes 7 and 17 | Hypovascular Multifocal | Less aggressive on average |
| Chromophobe RCC | Loss of chromosomes 1, 2, 6, 10, 13, 17, and 21 | Relatively hypovascular | Less aggressive on average |

**Hypervascular**

Increased number of blood vessels supplying a tumor. Kidney cancer is typically hypervascular due to the high expression of the growth factor VEGF.

**Multifocal**

Refers to having more than one tumor. Multifocal kidney cancer does not appear to be associated with worse prognosis, but can be a sign of an inherited kidney cancer.

**Satellite lesion**

Smaller tumors that grow near, but separate from the main renal cancer within the same kidney.

**Chromophobe renal cell carcinoma**

An uncommon type of kidney cancer responsible for less than 5% of kidney cancers. Most of these tumors do not spread outside of the kidney.

**Gene**

A segment of DNA that typically encodes a specific protein. Each gene contains an ordered sequence of the four nucleotides (A, C, G, and T).

The third most common type of kidney cancer is known as **chromophobe RCC**. These variants represent about 3–5% of all kidney cancers. Mutations include loss of a variety of chromosomes, but the exact **genes** involved are still under study. Like papillary RCC, these tumors tend to be less aggressive than clear cell RCC, but a small minority can behave in an aggressive manner.

Several other types of kidney cancer have been described, including collecting duct and **medullary cell**, and some kidney tumors appear so bizarre microscopically and genetically that they are termed "unclassified." In general, these other variants tend to behave in an aggressive manner, but some variant cancers can act less aggressively as well. Advanced molecular testing can help to better define these unusual cancers, but these techniques are still largely experimental and can't be relied on with 100% confidence at the present time.

## 7. What causes kidney cancer?

Kidney cancer, like all cancers, can be **inherited** or environmental. Inherited means that certain mutated genes that cause kidney cancer are passed down from generation to generation.

Inherited cancers are also known as **familial** kidney cancers, because they run in families.

Only about 3–4% of kidney cancers are familial, while the rest are believed to be **sporadic**. Sporadic refers to cancers that develop in an unpredictable manner in patients with no family history of kidney cancer. Familial kidney cancer tends to develop early in life and these patients tend to develop multiple tumors in the kidneys.

They can also develop tumors in other areas of the body, including the brain, spinal cord, and pancreas. Familial kidney cancer patients usually have relatives with a history of kidney cancer, and this is often one of the major clues to this diagnosis. Familial kidney cancer and particularly the **von Hippel-Lindau (VHL) syndrome**, is discussed in greater detail in the next few sections.

If the cancer is environmental it means that there has been exposure to carcinogens (cancer-causing substances) from, for example, smoking, the workplace, or one's diet. Carcinogens do their damage by mutating genes. If the gene that is mutated is in the kidney and is important for controlling cell growth, the kidney cell can then divide in an uncontrolled manner. This often occurs in a haphazard manner and additional mutations can then be generated. Eventually the tumor cells may become malignant and begin to divide uncontrollably. Of all the potential carcinogens, the one that is best proven is tobacco use, which increases the risk of developing kidney cancer by a factor of 2 to 3. If an individual stops smoking, this will eventually lead to a reduction in this risk over the next several years. Various chemicals that are used in certain industries, such as aromatic hydrocarbons, have also been suspected to cause kidney cancer, but in most cases this is not well proven.

Other environmental factors can increase the likelihood of developing kidney cancer. Studies from the United States and Europe have consistently shown obesity to put people at higher risk of developing kidney cancer. The typical high-fat and high-protein Western diet on which most Americans are raised may play a role in increasing the risk of kidney cancer, while a diet rich in fruits and vegetables may reduce this risk. High blood pressure and medications to lower the blood pressure may

**Medullary cell carcinoma**

An aggressive kidney cancer that occurs almost exclusively in patients with sickle cell trait or disease. Therefore, younger African Americans are most often affected.

**Inherited**

To receive (a characteristic) from one's parents by genetic transmission.

**Familial**

Occurring in the members of a family: a familial disease.

**Sporadic**

Occurring at random or by chance, and not as a result of a genetically determined, or inherited, trait.

**von Hippel-Lindau syndrome (VHL)**

A genetic disease caused by mutation of a tumor suppressor gene that has been called the VHL gene. Mutation of this gene is the most common cause of familial kidney cancer and also occurs in the majority of noninherited clear cell RCC.

also increase the risk of kidney cancer, but, like most of the factors mentioned here (with the exception of smoking), a direct link has not been established. **Radiation therapy** has also been implicated as a potential cause of kidney cancer in certain patients. Overall, the three most well-established, common risk factors for kidney cancer are tobacco use, hypertension, and obesity.

**Radiation therapy**

Treatment of disease by means of X-rays or radioactive substances.

## 8. Is kidney cancer inherited?

About 3–4% of kidney cancers are inherited. These cancers are known as familial because they run in families. A mutated gene in these families causes kidney cancer that is passed down from generation to generation. Since each person has two copies of each gene, the chance that the offspring will get the mutated gene is 50/50 (**autosomal dominant inheritance**). Persons having this gene are at substantially increased risk for developing kidney cancer, but this is not an all-or-nothing phenomenon.

**Autosomal dominant**

A pattern of inheritance in which half of the offspring will receive the mutated gene and develop the syndrome possessed by the parent.

The mutated genes allow the cells to divide in an uncontrolled manner leading to tumors. Every cell in the body carries the mutation so there are often several tumors in each kidney, and in some of the familial syndromes, tumors can also develop in other organs such as the brain and eyes. Another characteristic of familial cases is that kidney cancers are found early in life, in the 20s, 30s, or 40s, which is earlier than in cases of sporadic kidney cancer. In younger patients with kidney cancer, familial cancer is often suspected, and a family history of kidney cancer is sometimes, but not always, found.

# 9. What is the VHL syndrome?

VHL is short for von Hippel-Lindau syndrome, one of the familial syndromes of kidney cancer. In this syndrome, patients are born with a mutation of a gene on chromosome 3. Not surprisingly, this mutated gene has been named the von Hippel-Lindau gene, after the doctors who described the syndrome. Mutation of this gene places patients at risk for developing kidney cancer along with tumors of the eyes, the brain and spinal cord, and the adrenal glands. The **adrenal glands** are the glands that secrete **adrenaline** and are involved in response to stress. All of these tumors tend to be very vascular—they have great blood flow in and out of the tumor.

In these patients, the VHL gene mutation is present in all of the cells of the body, and tumors can also develop in other organs including the pancreas and inner ear. Typically, any given patient will develop only some of these tumor types—it is uncommon for a VHL patient to develop all of these cancers. As illustrated in **Table 2**, even kidney cancer, one of the hallmark tumors, is found in only about 24–70% of patients with this syndrome. All kidney tumors in patients with VHL are clear cell tumors.

Patients with VHL tend to develop kidney tumors very early in life, often in their 20s or 30s, and many patients will develop several kidney tumors in the course of their lifetime. Most of these tumors are small and nonaggressive, but some of the larger ones can metastasize. In fact, kidney cancer is the most common cause of death in this syndrome, so careful management of the kidney tumors is of paramount importance. The general consensus is to treat these tumors with surgical removal or **thermal ablation** (**cryoablation** or **radiofrequency ablation**) once they approach 3 cm in size or greater.

**Adrenal glands**

A small gland located on top of the kidney. The adrenal glands produce hormones that help control heart rate, blood pressure, the way the body uses food, the levels of minerals such as sodium and potassium in the blood, and other functions particularly involved in stress reactions.

**Adrenaline**

A hormone secreted by the adrenal glands that helps the body meet the demands of physical or emotional stress.

**Thermal ablation**

Destruction of a tumor using heat or cold to disrupt the cancer cells and blood vessels.

**Cryoablation**

Refers to destruction of a tumor by superfreezing. This procedure can be performed either under laparoscopic guidance or with radiographic guidance without the need for surgery. Also known as cryosurgical ablation, cryotherapy, or "cryo."

**Radiofrequency ablation**

An energy-based technology that uses alternating current to heat tissue, thereby causing direct cell death and injury and destruction of the tumor's blood supply.

**Nephrectomy**

Surgical removal of a kidney.

**Ophthalmologist**

A medical doctor specializing in the diagnosis and treatment of diseases of the eye.

Partial **nephrectomy** or other techniques that save as much kidney as possible are preferred in an effort to keep these patients off of dialysis as long as possible.

VHL is transmitted in an *autosomal dominant* manner: half of the children of an individual with the disease will receive the mutated gene and develop the disease. Most VHL patients have a family history of kidney cancer, brain or eye tumors, or blindness. If this syndrome is suspected, the patient should be evaluated for all of the other possible major manifestations of VHL, including a CT or MRI of the brain and spinal cord and referral to an **ophthalmologist**. **Genetic counseling** should also be considered and family members should be notified that they may be at risk and should be evaluated.

**Table 2** Familial Kidney Cancer Syndromes

| Syndrome | Mutation | Major Findings |
|---|---|---|
| VHL (von Hippel-Lindau) | VHL tumor suppressor gene (chromosome 3) | Clear cell RCC<br>Brain and spinal cord tumors<br>Eye tumors<br>Tumors of the adrenal glands |
| Hereditary Papillary Renal Cell Carcinoma | C-Met proto-onco-gene (chromosome 7) | Papillary RCC (multiple, often innumerable) |
| Familial Lieomytomatosis | Fumarate Hydratase (chromosome 1) | Papillary RCC (often aggressive)<br>Benign skin tumors<br>Uterine fibroids (leiomyomas)<br>Uterine leiomyosarcomas |
| Birt-Hogg-Dubé | Folliculin, from the BHD1 gene (chromosome 17) | Chromophobe RCC<br>Benign kidney tumors (oncocytoma)<br>Benign skin tumors<br>Lung cysts (fluid filled cavities)<br>Collapsed lung (pneumothorax) |

Table 3 shows several familial kidney cancer syndromes. Each has its own distinct genetic mutation and characteristic manner of presentation. Sophisticated genetic testing is available for each of these syndromes.

## 10. What is a tumor suppressor gene?

The VHL gene that is mutated in the von Hippel-Lindau syndrome is a tumor suppressor gene. A **tumor suppressor gene** encodes a protein that prevents the cell from dividing out of control—it acts like a brake on the cell to keep the cell in line (**Figure 2a**). Loss or malfunction of this brake is caused by mutation of the gene, causing the protein that is produced to stop functioning properly.

**Genetic counseling**

The counseling of individuals with established or potential genetic problems. This specialty is concerned with inheritance patterns and risks to other related family members, such as siblings and children.

**Tumor suppressor gene**

A gene that codes for a protein that serves to regulate cell division and prevent cancer growth. When the gene is mutated so that the protein is either not made or cannot function, tumor growth is able to proceed in an uncontrolled manner.

**Table 3** Tumors Found in the von Hippel-Lindau Syndrome of Familial Kidney Cancer

| Organ System | Lesion | Incidence |
|---|---|---|
| Eye | Benign retinal tumors (angioma) | 49–59% |
| Central nervous system (brain and spinal cord) | Benign vascular tumors (hemangiomas) | 42–72% |
| Kidney | Clear cell kidney cancer | 24–70% |
| | Kidney cysts (benign fluid filled cavities) | 22–59% |
| Adrenal gland | Pheochromocytoma (benign tumor that secretes adrenaline) | 18% |
| Pancreas | Benign tumors (islet cell tumors) | 12% |
| | Malignant tumors (islet cell tumors) | 2% |
| Epididymis | Benign tumors (cystadenoma) | 10–26% |
| Ear | Benign tumors (endolymphatic sac tumor) | 10% |

**Allele**

Any of the possible forms in which a gene for a specific trait can occur.

In reality, we are all born with two copies (or **alleles**) of every gene and both must be mutated before production of the protein ceases and the syndrome develops. However, in VHL patients, every cell in the kidney already has one mutated copy of the gene. The mutation has been passed on by one of the parents. Each cell is thus already half of the way toward losing the tumor suppressor protein. As the body's cells slowly divide to replace other cells that are naturally dying, the other copy may become mutated. In a normal person this would not be a problem because they have two normal copies and losing one is "covered up" by the other normal copy. But in VHL patients the other copy is already mutated. Each kidney has millions of cells and even with a low mutation rate, some will develop a mutation in the second VHL gene. These cells have then lost the

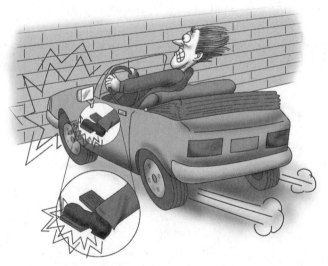

**Figure 2a** Tumor Suppressors. Cell division is under tight regulation by many pathways within the cell. Some genes prevent normal cell growth from spiraling out of control. These "tumor suppressors" act like a car's brakes. When tumor suppressor genes are mutated, it's as if the car brakes no longer function.

Reprinted with permission, Cleveland Clinic Center for Medical Art & Photography
© 2007–2014. All Rights Reserved.

tumor suppressor function, the brake, and can progress to cancer. This typically happens in several cells in the kidney, and this is the reason that patients with VHL typically form multiple kidney tumors.

Patients with sporadic (non-familial) clear cell kidney cancer typically will develop only a single tumor and this tends to happen later in life, in their 50s, 60s, or 70s. These patients, who represent the majority of kidney cancer patients, must mutate both copies of the VHL tumor suppressor gene in order to develop kidney cancer. Since the mutation rate of this gene is low, it is extremely unlikely that both copies in the same cell will be mutated. Even when this happens it tends to take a long time for this unfortunate event to occur. This explains why most patients with sporadic kidney cancer typically develop only one cancer and they tend to do so later in life.

In the end, the VHL tumor suppressor gene is directly involved in the formation of clear cell kidney cancer for both patients with sporadic cancer and those with the VHL familial syndrome, although the genetic pathways are different as highlighted above. Study of VHL families has been very important because it has allowed scientists to hone in on this gene, to localize it to chromosome 3, and eventually to completely sequence and characterize the gene and its protein product. Current studies are further clarifying the role that VHL plays in normal cells and cancer in order to identify pathways that can be targeted with new therapies for these patients.

## 11. What is an oncogene?

An **oncogene** is a mutation that activates a cell and transforms it into a cancer. An activated oncogene is

**Oncogene**

An oncogene is a mutation that activates a cell and transforms it into a cancer. An activated oncogene is analogous to having the accelerator of a car stuck in the "on position", the cell then divides out of control, gathers other mutations, and becomes malignant.

**Analogous**

Having similar function but a different structure and origin.

**analogous** to having the accelerator of a car stuck in the "on position"—the cell divides out of control, gathers other mutations, and becomes malignant (**Figure 2b**). One example of an oncogene is the C-Met gene that is mutated in hereditary papillary kidney cancer patients. This gene is passed down to half of the offspring—it is autosomal dominant. The protein that this gene encodes is a receptor for a growth factor. Normally, this receptor is activated only when exposed to certain growth factors, so the cell divides only during specific times. The mutation of this oncogene leaves the receptor active all of the time—it is stuck in the "on position." Oncogenes and tumor suppressor genes are mutated in a wide variety of cancers. Some of the oncogenes and tumor suppressor genes that are important for kidney cancer are now known, but it is likely that additional ones will be discovered in the future. Finding these mutations has

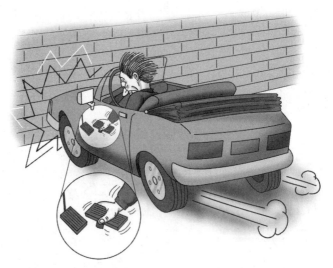

**Figure 2b** Oncogenes. When oncogenes are mutated (activated), they lead to uncontrolled cell growth which leads to cancer, like having a car's accelerator stuck in overdrive.

allowed us to reverse their action and has led to the development of exciting new treatments for patients with kidney cancer.

## 12. What is angiogenesis?

Tumors must stimulate the in-growth of new blood vessels to supply them with nutrients and oxygen. This is essential for a tumor to grow larger than 5 mm in size—otherwise, the center of the tumor will starve and die. The new blood vessels also provide the cancer cells with access to the bloodstream and are thus important for tumor cells to metastasize to other parts of the body. This process of new blood vessel growth is known as angiogenesis (**Figure 3**). Tumor cells secrete growth factors that stimulate angiogenesis, and this is regulated to some extent by various mutations that the cancer has acquired. For instance, clear cell tumors commonly have mutations in the VHL gene, and this leads to increased production of **vascular endothelial growth factor** (VEGF), an important growth factor that stimulates angiogenesis. Angiogenesis is very prominent in kidney cancer, particularly the clear cell type, and these cells become dependent on their new blood supply. Treatments that block angiogenesis by attacking these blood vessels have become available in the United States over the past several years. These anti-angiogenesis treatments, which include the FDA-approved drugs Sutent (sunitinib), Nexavar (sorafenib), Votrient (pazopanib), Inlyta (axitinib), and Avastin (bevacizumab) (see **Part Nine**), can partially starve a kidney cancer and slow its growth. They do this in part by blocking the action of VEGF. Compared to other treatments available for patients with advanced kidney cancer, these new treatments appear to be very promising (**Table 4**).

**Vascular endothelial growth factor (VEGF)**

A protein that is made within cells and released into the local environment. When cancer cells release VEGF, it stimulates the growth of new blood vessels, a process called angiogenesis. Although VEGF is just one of many factors that function in this way, it appears to play the major role in kidney cancer (and many other types of cancer).

*21*

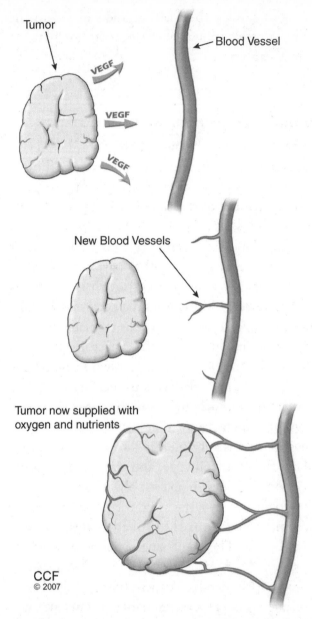

Tumor

Blood Vessel

VEGF

VEGF

VEGF

New Blood Vessels

Tumor now supplied with oxygen and nutrients

CCF
© 2007

**Figure 3** Angiogenesis is the process by which new blood vessels grow toward a tumor in order to provide it with oxygen and nutrients for additional growth. As a cancer grows, it makes substances like VEGF that encourage blood vessel cells to divide, sprout, and grow in its direction.

**Table 4** Treatments for Advanced Kidney Cancer and Treatment Mechanism

| Treatment | Mechanism | Common Uses |
|---|---|---|
| Surgery | Direct removal of the cancer or removal of the cancer that has not responded to other treatments | Removal of the kidney tumor is often combined with other systemic treatments; the goal of surgery in this setting is to debulk the cancer. Metasteses can be surgically removed if they are solitary or limited either before or after systemic treatments have been used |
| Radiation therapy | Radiation preferentially kills cancer cells | Only used if painful metastases to the bones<br><br>Can only treat a single or a few areas of the body |
| Chemotherapy | Most work by "poisoning" the cells, damaging DNA; preferentially tends to kill cancer cells | Still being investigated to try to find a chemotherapy regimen that might work better for kidney cancer, but success rates have been low (4–5% response rates) |
| Immunotherapy | Immunotherapy: works by activating the immune system to fight off the cancer | Commonly used until recently, high dose IL-2 is still considered by many to be the best chance for a cure, but even with this complete remissions are only seen in about 5% of patients<br><br>Overall response rates (complete remissions + partial responses) with immunotherapy are only 15–20%<br><br>Other approaches, such as inhibition of checkpoint control, are showing great promise |
| Anti-angiogenesis | Block the blood vessels that supply the tumor, and hence "starves" the tumor and slows its growth | Now commonly used for patients with advanced kidney cancer, includes treatments that inactivate VEGF or block the action of VEGF<br><br>40% response rates in some studies<br><br>Prolongs survival of many patients with kidney cancer<br><br>Not curative in most cases |

## 13. What is VEGF?

VEGF stands for vascular endothelial growth factor. This is a protein that acts as a growth factor that stimulates angiogenesis. It is secreted by kidney cancers and acts on nearby blood vessels by stimulating them to sprout new blood vessels. These new blood vessels then grow into the tumor and supply it with nutrients and oxygen, enabling the tumor to continue to grow and expand. The secretion of VEGF by kidney cancer cells is regulated by the VHL tumor suppression gene. When this gene is mutated, as it commonly is in clear cell kidney cancer, the cancer cells increase their secretion of this growth factor. VEGF acts on receptors on the surface of blood vessel cells. These receptors transmit a signal into the blood vessel cells, causing them to divide and reorganize to form new blood vessels.

**Antibodies**

Proteins in the blood that are produced by the body in response to specific foreign proteins (such as those made by bacteria). Antibodies then trigger the immune system to respond to the foreign proteins.

Most of the new and exciting treatments for kidney cancer target VEGF, either by using **antibodies** (Avastin® [bevacimuzab]—see Question 78) to bind and inactivate VEGF or by blocking the receptors for VEGF. In the latter case, drugs like Sutent® (sunitinib—see Question 79) and Nexavar® (sorafenib—see Question 79) act primarily by inhibiting the receptors that detect VEGF and send its signal inside the cell. Therefore, they make the blood vessel cells insensitive to the effects of VEGF. VEGF is thus a key factor regulating the growth of kidney cancer and angiogenesis related to this cancer.

## 14. Can kidney cancer be prevented?

The total number of kidney cancers would be substantially reduced if no one used tobacco products—no cigarettes, no cigars, and no tobacco chewing. This would be the single best way to reduce the incidence and mortality rates related to this cancer, and the same is clearly true for many other cancers including lung cancer, throat cancer, and bladder cancer. In addition, most healthcare professionals believe that a healthy diet and good weight control will reduce the risk of many cancers, including kidney cancer. Recent studies indicate that 20% and 30% of all kidney cancers can be attributed to tobacco and obesity, respectively. High-fat and high-protein intake appear to increase the risk of developing kidney cancer, while increased fruit and vegetable consumption may decrease this risk. Daily vitamins have not been well studied with respect to possibly reducing the risk of kidney cancer, so we do not know whether vitamins will help.

Although the rates of kidney cancer can be reduced on a population-wide level by adopting healthy practices, most cases of sporadic kidney cancer (i.e., cancer in people with no family history) are related to unfortunate mutations that are not likely to be preventable. Each time the cell divides, it must duplicate the **DNA** contained on each of its **chromosomes** and this requires very precise realignment of the genetic code. Inevitably, occasional errors are made when aligning the more than three billion base pairs of DNA that code for the 50,000–100,000 genes in each person's complete set of genes (**genome**).

Fortunately, most of these mutations are masked by a normal second allele (we all have two copies or alleles of each gene). However, on occasion both alleles may become affected or one dominant mutation will predominate. If this affects a gene that regulates important cellular functions, such as the VHL gene, a cancer may develop. Most of the time, these mutations cannot be attributed to a specific cause that we can currently identify, and to some extent is just bad luck.

**DNA**

Also known as deoxyribonucleic acid. DNA is the building block of the genes that encode for each of the proteins present in the body's cells. Each gene contains an ordered sequence of the four nucleotides and are comprised of matched pairs of nucleotides (A with T, C with G, etc.) and the two strands of DNA (A, adenine; C, cytosine; G, guanine; T, thymine).

**Chromosome**

All of a person's genes (genome) are encoded on 23 pairs of chromosomes. Each chromosome consists of two intertwined strands of DNA wrapped around a protein core.

**Genome**

The total amount of genetic information in the chromosomes of an organism, including its genes and DNA sequences. The human genome is made up of about 50,000–100,000 genes.

Hence, most cases of kidney cancer are not preventable, but are an inevitable result of an increasingly aging population. As we get older we gradually accumulate mutations as the years pass by. Our risk of developing kidney cancer, as well as other cancers, continues to increase as we age. The average person prior to the 1900s only lived until about 50 to 60 years of age and commonly died from heart disease, infections, or other medical causes. In those days most people died before they reached the age that cancer would become an issue. With the increasing life expectancy of people in the United States and around the world, cancer is becoming a problem of epidemic proportion.

Patient—Cheryl S.:

*Looking back on what I could have done to possibly prevent my kidney cancer would be to not smoke and to exercise on a routine basis with a healthy diet.*

## 15. Are all kidney cancers aggressive?

Some kidney cancers are aggressive and can spread (or metastasize) to other parts of the body. These cancers often will not respond adequately to our current treatments and may eventually lead to the death of the patient. They occasionally do this by hindering essential bodily functions such as blocking the bowels or replacing enough of the lungs that the patient can no longer breathe effectively, but more commonly they just lead to a state of generalized weakness and **malnutrition** that eventually leads to death. Eventually, a patient with advanced cancer becomes too weak to sustain life. These are the cancers that account for the estimated 13,000 kidney cancer-related deaths in the United States each year.

**Malnutrition**

Lack of proper nutrition; inadequate or unbalanced nutrition.

Many other kidney cancers are less aggressive and are diagnosed before they acquire or express these aggressive tendencies. These tumors actually account for about two-thirds of all kidney cancers, and this is fortunate because these patients can be cured of the cancer. These tumors are confined to the kidney and can be surgically removed, either with **partial nephrectomy** or **radical nephrectomy**. Many of these tumors are small, but even some very large tumors can be cured surgically if they are still confined to the kidney.

In general, clear cell tumors are more aggressive than the other major subtypes (papillary and chromophobe). However, the majority of clear cell tumors are confined to the kidney and are, therefore, surgically curable. Most papillary or chromophobe tumors are also confined, but a small minority (5–10%) can behave in an aggressive manner. Other factors that can provide an indication of the aggressive potential of a kidney cancer include the **tumor grade** (how aggressive the cancer cells look under the microscope), tumor size (larger tumors are more likely to be aggressive), and whether the patient was diagnosed with symptoms or incidentally (no symptoms).

All of these factors give us a hint as to aggressive potential but none are "all or nothing." Many kidney tumors are now being diagnosed incidentally in patients with an upset stomach or other nonspecific abdominal symptoms. These patients undergo a CT scan or ultrasound to try to detect a possible cause of their discomfort and are found to have a kidney tumor. Many of these are small (< 4 cm size) and these tumors are variable in terms of their aggressive potential. About 20% of these tumors are benign, 60% are malignant but relatively slow growing, and 20% are malignant and have the potential for more aggressive behavior. Ideally, this

**Partial nephrectomy**

Removal of the portion of the kidney that contains the tumor, along with just enough healthy kidney to provide a safe margin.

**Radical nephrectomy**

The surgical removal of a kidney, usually performed in the treatment of cancer of the kidney.

**Tumor grade**

Tumor grade is a way of classifying tumors based on certain features of their cells. The grade of a tumor is directly linked to prognosis. Using a microscope, a pathologist studies the tumor tissue removed during a biopsy to check: 1) How much the cancer cells look like normal cells. (The more the cancer cells look like normal cells, the lower the tumor grade tends to be.) 2) How many of the cancer cells are in the process of dividing (The fewer cancer cells that are in the process of dividing, the more likely it is that the tumor is slow-growing and the lower the tumor grade tends to be.) Together, these two factors determine the tumor grade.

would be sorted out prior to surgery, but typical radiographic studies (CT, MRI, ultrasound) do not provide this information and biopsies are not always accurate enough—sometimes they indicate that a malignant tumor is benign, or vice versa. Biopsy can be performed if the results will change the type of treatment selected, such as avoiding surgery for a definite diagnosis of a benign tumor or performing surgery for a cancer in a patient with elevated surgical risks that might otherwise have his or her tumor observed.

Therefore, most patients will be treated based on the results of their **radiographic tests**: if the X-rays suggest that a lesion is probably a cancer, then they need to be treated with the presumption that it is a cancer. Most of these tumors are treated with surgery, which provides an accurate diagnosis and best chance for cure.

**Radiographic tests**

An examination performed to visualize parts of the body that are not visible with the naked eye. These tests use some form of energy to "see" a person's insides. Common types include plain X-ray, tomography (CT), magnetic resonance imaging (MRI), and ultrasound (US).

Patient—Cheryl S.:

*I had a very large tumor and had lymph node involvement outside of my one kidney. My physician was able to save 55% of my functioning kidney and I am cancer free today!*

## 16. Should we be screening the general population for kidney cancer?

Patients often wonder whether their cancer could have been found sooner and whether their doctor should have done a screening test for a given type of cancer. An ideal screening test would be simple, inexpensive, exquisitely accurate, and widely available. For certain cancers, such as colorectal cancer, an excellent screening test exists and has been recommended by the United States Agency for Healthcare Research and Quality. Colonoscopy is a test that can detect cancers and precancerous lesions within the bowels, which can also often be removed during the procedure. Current recommendations are that anyone 50 years of age or older should undergo colonoscopy as a screening test, and then have the test repeated fairly frequently if colon polyps are found. This approach can lead to the early diagnosis of colon cancer and has been demonstrated to reduce the death rate from this cancer; unfortunately not everyone who should have a colonoscopy chooses to have one performed. Colon cancer is a relatively common cancer and one of the most lethal, accounting for about 10% of cancer-related deaths in the United States, thus screening patients makes sense.

The rationale behind screening for kidney cancer is that it might lead to earlier detection when the cancer is still confined and able to be removed surgically. In reality, this is the only circumstance for which a high cure rate can be expected. Based on this, screening for kidney cancer has been studied through the use of ultrasound to visualize the kidneys. Ultrasound is an appealing study for screening purposes because it is virtually painless and risk free. It works by sending out sound waves and detecting their reflection off of the internal organs. It is analogous to sonar used to detect submarines. However, the studies that have been done have shown that only a very small number of kidney cancers are detected in this manner because the incidence of this cancer is so low. For instance, if you screened 100,000 people, only about 50 kidney tumors would be found, a relatively small number for such cancer screening studies. Some of the 50 tumors would be benign or indolent (nonaggressive) and you would be making a difference in terms of survival for only a few patients. The cost would be exorbitant (each ultrasound would cost $100–$500), and given the high costs of health care in our country today this would not be supportable. To put it in simple terms, until a more affordable screening tool is discovered, the money is better spent elsewhere.

Another way to screen for kidney cancer would be to look for blood in the urine using a microscope or a dipstick, taking advantage of the fact that blood in the urine is one of the major warning signs for kidney cancer. However, this type of screening would miss many cancers, because many kidney tumors, especially the smaller, contained tumors, do not spill blood into the urine. Once again, there is the inescapable issue of the cost of this type of screening.

At this point in time, we cannot justify general screening for kidney cancer. Perhaps there will come a day when our "stethoscopes" will enable each internist to quickly and inexpensively scan the internal organs of every patient to look for kidney cancer, pancreatic cancer, aortic aneurysms, and a variety of other disorders. Unfortunately, we are not there yet. In the meantime, we should focus our screening efforts primarily on populations with an increased risk of kidney cancer, so called "target populations."

## 17. Who is at highest risk for developing kidney cancer?

Everyone has a small risk of developing kidney cancer. One out of every 10,000 adults in America will be diagnosed with this cancer each year. But some groups have a higher risk of developing kidney cancer. These groups are known as "target populations," and screening in these groups of people should be considered. Target populations for kidney cancer include:

- Patients with known VHL or other familial kidney cancer syndromes, or direct relatives of such patients. Patients with VHL or other familial forms of kidney cancer should have a CT or ultrasound at least every other year, as well as screening for other tumors that can develop in these syndromes. Relatives should consider genetic analysis to see if they harbor the mutated gene; if so, they should also be followed closely as outlined above.

- Patients with end-stage renal disease commonly develop cysts (fluid-filled cavities) and about 1% will also subsequently develop kidney cancer. Three years after starting on dialysis or undergoing kidney transplant, patients that are still relatively young and healthy should undergo a screening ultrasound or CT and then periodically thereafter.

- Patients with tuberous sclerosis, a syndrome in which patients develop benign skin lesions, vascular lesions in the brain that can cause seizures or mental retardation, benign vascular lesions in the kidneys (**angiomyolipomas**), and kidney cancer. These patients should undergo screening ultrasound or CT periodically, presuming that they are otherwise healthy and have a good quality of life.

**Angiomyolipoma**
A benign tumor composed of fat tissue, muscle cells, and vascular structures.

At some time in the future, we will be able to take a small blood sample and conduct a sophisticated molecular genetic analysis that will give us a good estimation of each person's risk for each of the common and important cancers, and this will guide our decisions with regard to screening for various cancers. However, we are not there yet. Until then, we will need to focus our screening efforts primarily on the target populations mentioned previously. If you would like to speed up progress in this field, and have the resources, please consider donating money for cancer research.

## 18. Should my family members be evaluated for kidney cancer?

Cancer patients often wonder whether their relatives are at risk and need to be evaluated. For kidney cancer, most of the time the answer is no. The typical patient with kidney cancer has sporadic disease and no prior family history of this type of malignancy. They typically have a solitary tumor and tend to present later in life—older than 55 years of age. These patients represent greater than 90% of all patients with kidney cancer. The chance that their relatives will develop kidney cancer is still very low and routine evaluation or screening is not recommended. On the other hand, the blood relatives of patients with familial kidney cancer should be evaluated because they may be at elevated risk of developing kidney cancer. If the family member with kidney cancer has a known genetic mutation, she/he should consider genetic testing to learn whether she/he also carries the mutated gene. If so, she/he should be evaluated with an ultrasound or CT to look for kidney cancer. Other testing may also be required depending on the circumstances. This proactive approach will often lead to early diagnosis and can be lifesaving.

Hints that a person with kidney cancer may have familial kidney cancer can include:

- Prior family history of kidney cancer, kidney failure of unknown origin, eye tumors, blindness, and spinal or brain tumors
- Early age of onset of kidney cancer
- Multifocal disease (multiple kidney tumors)
- Association of kidney cancer with adrenal tumors, pancreatic tumors, visual problems or eye tumors, or brain or spinal cord tumors

• Association with other manifestations of the various syndromes, as outlined in Tables 2 and 3 in Question 9.

In these settings, familial kidney cancer should be considered and screening or evaluation of the other family members should be discussed.

## 19. Is kidney cancer seen in children?

Kidney cancer is uncommon in children. Most kidney tumors that are detected in children are **Wilms' tumors**, a different type of cancer that is seen primarily in children. This tumor is often treated with a combination of surgery and chemotherapy, and occasionally with radiation therapy. For most children with Wilms' tumors, survival rates are good, but some patients with advanced disease do not do well. Classic kidney cancer, also known as renal cell carcinoma, is also seen in children, but is much less common. These tumors have been shown to possess unique mutations that affect the TFE3 gene that is likely responsible for the tumors that develop at such a young age. Kidney cancer in children and young adults is more likely to be high grade and locally advanced, but many of these children will do well with an aggressive treatment approach that combines surgical removal and systemic treatments.

**Wilms' tumor**

A malignant kidney tumor occurring in young children and composed of small spindle cells and other tissue.

## 20. Are men or women more likely to have kidney cancer?

Overall, 60% of kidney cancers are seen in men and 40% in women. There does not appear to be a major difference in terms of the aggressive potential between cancers detected in either gender. However, one difference is that kidney tumors found in women are more likely to be benign, rather than a kidney cancer. This is particularly true for young or middle-aged women.

Again, not all tumors in the kidney that are found on imaging studies represent kidney cancer. Overall, about 80% are malignant and 20% are benign. Benign kidney tumors are more common (> 20%) in women, suggesting that they may be somehow related to hormonal changes that routinely occur with the menstrual cycle or with menopause. When we evaluate a young or middle-aged woman, we consider the possibility of a benign tumor, although the X-rays or biopsy often cannot pin this down with 100% certainty. Therefore, even these patients will require surgery, although doctors would try to perform a partial nephrectomy, if possible, because they would not want to remove the whole kidney if this could be avoided. Beyond this, there is very little difference between men and women when it comes to kidney cancer.

Caregiver—Linda C.:

*Kidney cancer is the disease that took my daughter from me, her four children, husband, father, and sister. My daughter did not fit the profile of a typical kidney cancer patient. She was a nonsmoking, 32-year-old woman who lived a healthy, active lifestyle. She was diagnosed 4 weeks after her fourth child was born. She complained of blood in her urine, fatigue, and lower back pain during her last trimester of pregnancy. After her baby was born, she contacted a urologist who immediately sent her for a CT scan. Her "severe kidney infection" turned out to be a tumor the size of a watermelon that weighed over 10 pounds (more than her baby). I cannot emphasize enough—no one knows your body like you do—if you are having health issues and your doctor disregards your symptoms, find a doctor who will listen! This is your life!*

## 21. Are other types of cancer seen in the kidney?

Since the kidney is a very vascular organ, other cancers that get into the bloodstream will pass through the kidneys and often find them to be fertile soil for setting up camp. Hence, the kidneys are one of the most common sites of metastasis for many types of cancer. Studies of autopsies in which patients dying of other cancers were examined from head to toe indicate that the kidney is near the top of the list of involved organs. The most common cancers to metastasize to the kidneys are lung cancer, breast cancer, colon cancer, and melanoma; however, any type of cancer can metastasize to the kidney. Common clues that a cancer in the kidney is not a kidney cancer, but rather a metastasis from another cancer include:

- The patient is known to have a cancer somewhere else in the body or has been treated for another cancer in the past.

- The appearance of the tumor(s) on radiographic studies is not typical. Metastases often have less blood flow than classic kidney cancer, and appear less vascular on a CT scan.

- Multiple tumors within the kidney, since fewer than 15% of patients with kidney cancer present with more than a single tumor. Metastases to the kidney are often multifocal.

In these settings, a biopsy will often be performed in order to determine whether a detected lesion is a kidney cancer or a metastasis to the kidney. Patients with metastatic disease to the kidney will likely not benefit from kidney surgery and may be offered systemic treatment based on the origin of the cancer.

# PART THREE

# Presentation and Evaluation

What are the typical signs and symptoms
of kidney cancer?

What is hematuria?

What kind of doctor should I be seeing?

*More*\*...

## 22. What are the typical signs and symptoms of kidney cancer?

The classic symptoms of kidney cancer include:

- **Hematuria,** or blood in the urine
- Abdominal pain, up in the area of the kidney, also known as the flank
- Palpable abdominal mass, meaning that the patient or doctor can feel the mass through the skin
- Weight loss, fevers, night sweats, fatigue and/ or other generalized symptoms that are known as constitutional since they reflect a weakened constitution
- **Paraneoplastic syndromes,** literally meaning syndromes that are found in association with a neoplasm, where the kidney cancer secretes proteins that circulate throughout the body and cause one or more of the following:
  - Hypercalcemia, or elevated blood levels of calcium. This is associated with weakness and fatigue, decreased reflexes, and altered mental status.
  - **Erythrocytosis,** where the red blood cell counts rise (the opposite of anemia). This can lead to blood clotting or thrombosis in severe cases.
  - Hypertension, related to secretion of a protein (**renin**) that drives the blood pressure up.
  - Liver malfunction, also known as Stauffer's syndrome.
- Symptoms directly due to metastasis, such as a chronic cough that is sometimes seen in patients with lung metastases or bony pain that can occur in patients with bone metastases

**Hematuria**

The presence of blood in the urine.

**Paraneoplastic syndrome**

A disorder caused by the release of certain compounds by the kidney cancer cells.

**Erythrocytosis**

An increase in red blood cell count numbers in the blood stream that can be seen in kidney cancer patients. It is thought to be due to increased production of a stimulant of red blood cell production, called erythropoietin.

**Renin**

A hormone of high specificity that is released by the kidney and acts to raise blood pressure by activating angiotensin.

In the modern era, most patients with kidney cancer are diagnosed in an asymptomatic state—they have no signs or symptoms of kidney cancer. The cancer is found during a computed tomography (CT) scan or ultrasound obtained for other purposes, which is known as incidental discovery. This is a good thing because any of the above signs or symptoms suggests an increased likelihood that the kidney cancer might be more serious or difficult to treat.

## 23. What is hematuria?

Hematuria, or blood in the urine, is a major warning sign of cancer in the urinary system, much like blood in the stool or coughing up blood are warning signs of other cancers. However, blood in the urine does not always signify cancer. It has a variety of causes including:

- Kidney or bladder cancer—these are the ones that we worry about most.

- Other cancers in this area of the body, such as tumors of the **ureters** or **urethra**.

- Kidney or bladder stones.

- Infections of the urinary tract, including infections of the bladder (**cystitis**), prostate (prostatitis), and kidneys (pyelonephritis).

- Trauma or injury to the urinary tract, often related to sports or motor vehicle accidents, but this is usually obvious and the patient will often recall a recent accident that may have been causative.

- Benign conditions, such as benign growth of the prostate or certain inflammatory lesions of the bladder or kidney.

**Ureters**

The paired structures that carry urine from each kidney to the bladder.

**Urethra**

The canal through which urine is discharged from the bladder.

**Cystitis**

Inflammation of the urinary bladder.

- Benign, but potentially serious conditions where the kidneys leak blood into the urine causing chronic kidney disease. Normally the filters of the kidneys will not allow blood cells to cross over into the urine, but in certain conditions, known as **glomerulonephritis,** this can happen.
- Benign vascular abnormalities of the kidneys or bladder.
- Blood thinners, which can increase the risk of bleeding into the urine. These patients should still be evaluated because they often have some underlying pathology that the blood thinners are allowing to become apparent.

**Glomerulonephritis**

A kidney disease affecting the small blood vessels of the glomeruli of the kidney, characterized by leakage of protein into the urine (albuminuria), fluid retention within the body(edema), and high blood pressure (hypertension).

Patients with blood in the urine, whether readily visible or microscopic, should undergo a focused evaluation to sort this out. This will typically require a blood test to check kidney function, some simple urine tests to look for infection or cancer cells, an X-ray study to look at the kidneys, and cystoscopy to look at the internal lining of the bladder. All of these tests are typically required to determine the cause in adults with hematuria.

Patient—Cheryl S.

*"I was urinating blood (hematuria) and went straight to my PCP and started an immediate investigation as to why that was occurring. I had blood work, scan of my bladder, and then a CT of my abdomen and that's when they found the tumor. In my lab work I had erythocytosis, where my blood cell count was abnormally high."*

## 24. What kind of doctor should I be seeing?

The type of doctor that you need is determined primarily by the stage of the cancer, but regardless of the stage, a **urologist** should be involved. Urologists specialize in diseases of the kidneys, bladder, prostate, and male reproductive organs. They are the surgeons for these areas of the body and are typically the main doctors for patients with kidney tumors. The urologist will direct the evaluation of a suspected kidney tumor and help to determine whether the tumor is benign or malignant. He or she will also determine what other tests are needed to stage the cancer and determine whether there are metastases (spread of the cancer).

If the tumor is associated with metastasis to other areas of the body, then a medical **oncologist** should also be involved in your care. Patients with advanced kidney cancer often need both surgery and systemic treatments, and both a urologist and a medical oncologist should be involved to coordinate these treatments.

Ideally, the doctors you see would have specialized training in urologic cancers, and in kidney cancer in particular. This helps them to know all of the ins and outs about this type of cancer. Such specialists often have access to clinical trials that may allow for progressive treatment **protocols**, in which patients can receive additional treatments if the cancer has not responded to initial treatments. Some of these trials offer promising new drugs that might not be available otherwise. In the modern era, a surgeon with minimally-invasive surgery experience should be considered, since radical nephrectomy, partial nephrectomy, and ablative techniques can now often be done with laparoscopic or robot-assisted

*The type of doctor that you need is determined primarily by the stage of the cancer.*

**Urologist**

A physician who specializes in urology, including the clinical, surgical, and scientific aspects of the genitourinary tract in health and disease.

**Oncologist**

A specialist in oncology, dealing with the diagnosis and medical treatment of cancer.

**Protocol**

The plan for a course of medical treatment or for a clinical trial.

laparoscopic techniques. These laparoscopic procedures (see Question 50) are typically associated with less post-operative pain and a more rapid recovery.

As always, an experienced, board-certified doctor with a good reputation is most desirable. Of course, a variety of other factors (e.g., bedside manner, ability to explain important aspects of the care) are also important. A second opinion can also be considered, particularly if there are any major questions or uncertainties after the initial evaluation.

Caregiver—Linda C.:

*Because chemo and radiation are not effective for most kidney cancer patients, I think it is very important that the kidney cancer patient be seen by a kidney cancer specialist. If distance is an issue, many times the renal cell carcinoma (RCC) specialist will work with your local oncologist. You want to be seen by someone who is experienced with this disease—someone who will give you hope and will be aggressive if the need arises.*

## 25. Does the type of hospital matter?

The type of hospital can make a difference for some patients and in certain circumstances. For instance, complex patients that not only have a kidney tumor, but also heart disease will often be best managed in a referral hospital. In this setting, top-notch cardiologists and anesthesiologists are available to help with the patient's care if needed. Streamlined coordination of care prior to and following surgery are important for obtaining the best results. Many laparoscopic and open kidney surgeries are complex and are best performed at a referral hospital, because some of these procedures are technically demanding and relatively high risk. These types of procedures are probably best performed by a doctor who does them routinely. In the end, the most important factor with these procedures is the experience and expertise of the surgeon(s) who will be involved in your care.

Complex patients with advanced kidney cancer who may require the latest clinical protocols may also be best served in a referral center, particularly one with a dedicated cancer center. Such centers are on the cutting edge of the field and often are participating in clinical trials that are not available at other hospitals. Some of these trials offer promising new drugs that might not be available otherwise.

## Patient—Dennis W.

*When I was diagnosed with renal cell carcinoma, my local physician said there were a few choices as to where I would receive treatment. We chose the institution where I was treated for several reasons. First and foremost was word of mouth—so many people told us of the great care they were given there. Second, many of the physicians we talked to recommended that treatment center. We have found it makes a difference where you choose to receive treatment. You should choose a treatment center that has the technology and staff to accommodate your needs.*

## Patient—Cheryl S.

*I obtained two different opinions due to the size of the tumor and the stage of my cancer. Find a physician that truly understands kidney cancer and who can perform the surgery, and understands all the new treatment options. Always do your part in looking for who you pick for a physician. Do a background check and don't be afraid to ask about outcomes with that doctor's patients. You truly need to trust your physician and have a great relationship with the office staff.*

## 26. What tests are usually performed?

The evaluation of patients with kidney cancer includes a careful history about potential symptoms and a physical examination, and then a number of tests are considered. These will usually include blood tests to check the complete blood counts (also known as a CBC) and to look at kidney and liver function and serum electrolytes (also known as a complete metabolic panel). Some centers also use C-reactive protein to monitor for kidney cancer, although this test can give a high reading in a number of other conditions, and is therefore not specific for cancer. A CT scan of the abdomen and pelvis is typically performed with contrast and is carefully reviewed to evaluate for local extension of the cancer or for lymph node involvement. Finally, a chest X-ray is done to look for possible lung metastases. For most patients with kidney cancer, this is the only testing that is required.

*The evaluation of patients with kidney cancer includes a careful history about potential symptoms and a physical examination.*

If you are considered high risk due to large tumor size or aggressive appearance of the tumor on a CT scan or if you have bone pain or other symptoms then other tests may be considered. This may include a bone scan, CT scan of the chest, or a CT or MRI scan of the brain. However, these tests are not needed in most patients. Finally, an MRI scan of the abdomen and pelvis is also occasionally required, particularly if there is concern about extension of the cancer into the major veins coming out of the kidney. This is not always seen well on the initial CT scan. MRI is also considered in patients with kidney failure, in whom a CT scan cannot be obtained safely because of the damage that **intravenous** contrast can cause to the kidneys. In addition, some patients may require additional testing to

**Intravenous**

Within or through the blood; usually refers to medications or fluids given through an IV line.

evaluate other medical conditions. For example, patients with symptoms suggestive of heart disease may need a stress test to evaluate their condition prior to surgery. To some extent, your doctor must tailor your evaluation to fit your individual situation.

## 27. What is an ultrasound?

Ultrasonography uses sound waves that are transmitted through the skin and into the body. These sound waves reflect off of the internal organs. The pattern of sound waves that is reflected back is then detected and this allows us to "visualize" the internal organs for any possible tumors or cysts. Ultrasound is very analogous to sonar that was used to detect submarines during World War II. Since this test relies on just sound waves, it is very safe and there is essentially no exposure to radiation. Side effects or complications related to ultrasonography are very uncommon.

The test is typically performed by a technician working under the supervision of a radiologist. A transducer is placed against the skin and acts as both the source and detector for the sound waves. The transducer is pushed gently against the skin overlying the kidneys and rotated in various directions to allow the kidneys to be visualized and evaluated. Each organ has its own characteristic "**echogenic** pattern" that can be readily identified. Disruption of this pattern by a solid tumor is usually relatively easy to recognize. Most kidney tumors have either increased or decreased echogenicity and will stand out against the background of the normal kidney (**Figure 4**).

**Echogenic**

The pattern of sound waves detected during an ultrasound examination. Kidney tumors can have increased or decreased echogenicity on ultrasound when compared to normal kidney. The main advantages of ultrasonography are that it is very safe and relatively inexpensive, but it often must be combined with other tests to yield a definitive diagnosis.

**Anechoic**

Not having or producing echoes. Used to describe cystic lesions on ultrasound, because they do not send back echoes.

Cysts, or fluid-filled cavities, are easily identified with ultrasound since they are water-filled and therefore **anechoic** (they do not reflect sound waves and thus appear as a black cavity). Most cysts are thin-walled and filled with water and these common cysts are known as simple cysts. They are benign and do not require further evaluation. If a cyst has irregular thick walls, is heavily calcified, or has blood within it, it will yield a more complex pattern on ultrasound and is considered a complex cyst. Some of these cysts are malignant and a CT scan or MRI is recommended for further characterization.

The main advantages of ultrasonography are that it is very safe and relatively inexpensive, but it often must be combined with other tests to yield a definitive diagnosis.

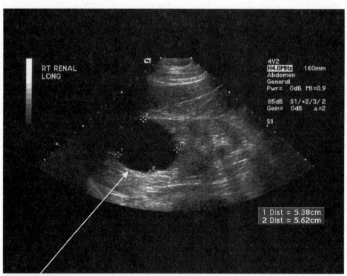

Simple Cyst

**Figure 4a** Appearance of renal lesions on ultrasound. Ultrasonic waves do not bounce back from a simple cyst, making it appear dark (hypoechoic) on ultrasound.

Also, ultrasonography is often inadequate in morbidly obese patients because the internal organs are further away from the skin and the sound waves become distorted by the fat.

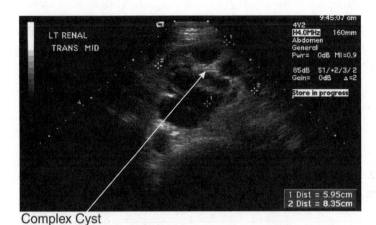

Complex Cyst

**Figure 4b** Complex cysts have internal divisions (septae) or other irregular features.

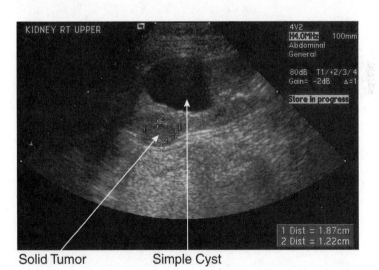

Solid Tumor          Simple Cyst

**Figure 4c** Simple cysts and complex cysts can usually be distinguished from a solid tumor on ultrasound because a tumor reflects more signal back to the probe than the cyst.

## 28. What is a CT scan?

CT scans are the most useful radiographic tests for the evaluation of kidney tumors (**Figure 5a**). During a CT scan the patient is brought through a cylindrical scanner that images the internal organs, and this information is stored on a computer (**Figure 5b**). The various images can then be reorganized and printed or just directly visualized on the computer. Each image shows a "slice of the body" and allows us to visualize the internal anatomy in all of its detail. The most common images are transverse or horizontal and show us exactly the anatomy at that level of the body.

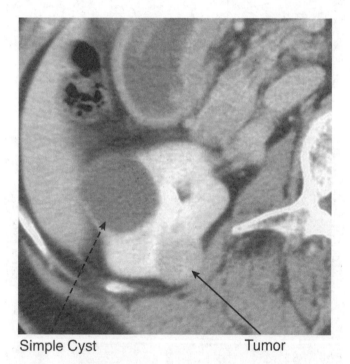

Simple Cyst                                    Tumor

**Figure 5a** Appearance of renal lesions on computed tomography (CT). CT scan of a renal cell carcinoma (solid arrow), which shows uptake of contrast within the kidney tumor (enhancement). Uptake of contrast suggests increased blood flow in and out of the tumor, and this indicates a high risk of malignancy. A simple cyst (water filled cavity) that does not enhance with contrast is also shown (dashed arrow).

Each subsequent image shows the next level of the body, just 3–10 mm below the first one, and so on. In this way, the entire body can be visualized. It is not an overstatement to say that CT scans have revolutionized modern medicine. You might wonder why we do not obtain CT scans more often, given their potential utility. CT scans entail a relatively high radiographic exposure and they are somewhat expensive; therefore, they should not be obtained indiscriminately. In fact, even for patients who need a CT scan, we will typically try to limit the study to the area of interest. For instance, for patients with a kidney tumor, often only the abdomen and pelvis is scanned, and the chest and brain are scanned only under special circumstances.

CT scans can sometimes tell us whether a tumor is benign or malignant because some benign kidney tumors have unique characteristics. For example, an

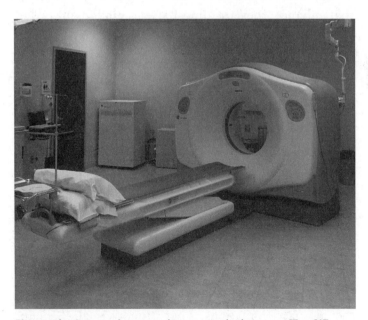

**Figure 5b** Computed tomography scanner, also known as CT or CAT scanner.

angiomyolipoma is a benign kidney tumor that has fat intermixed within the tumor, and in most cases this will declare itself on CT (**Figure 5c**). Then again other benign kidney tumors, such as oncocytomas, cannot be differentiated from kidney cancer since they look very similar with a CT scan. In general, tumors that "light up" after administration of intravenous contrast are more likely to be malignant because this reflects increased blood flow in and out of the tumor. Tumors that fail to enhance with contrast are likely to be benign—many are postinflammatory scar tissue, benign anatomic variants, or benign tumors. One useful rule of thumb is that any solid, enhancing renal mass that does not contain fat density must be considered a malignant kidney cancer and must be treated as such. When these are removed surgically, 80–90% prove to be malignant.

CT scans are also very useful for the evaluation of complex cysts of the kidney. If these cysts have nodular areas that enhance, they are almost always malignant. If they are water dense and thin-walled, they are simple cysts and are benign and do not require further evaluation (**Figure 5d**). If they have internal septations or divisions, are calcified, or contain blood from prior hemorrhage, the CT will visualize this and allow doctors to estimate the risk of malignancy.

CT scans will not only show a kidney tumor but they help your physician to stage the cancer. CT scans will show enlarged lymph nodes, extension into adjacent organs, or metastasis to other organs such as the liver or lungs. CT can also demonstrate invasion of the tumor into the venous system, although MRI is still considered the premier study for this. As powerful as CT scans are they do have limitations. They cannot visualize microscopic extension of cancer. Cancer within a lymph node

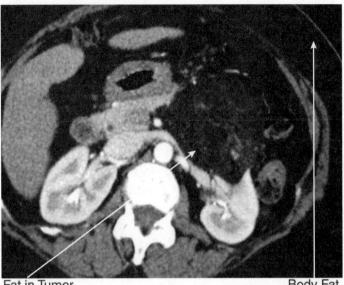

Fat in Tumor                                    Body Fat

**Figure 5c** CT can also distinguish some benign tumors of the kidney, such as angiomyolipoma, which contains fat. On this CT, the majority of this tumor has the same density (color) as the fat surrounding the abdomen.

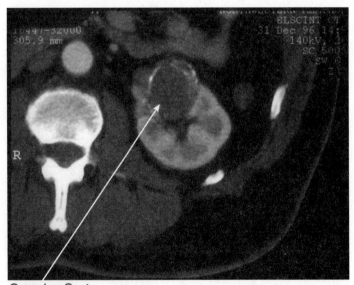

Complex Cyst

**Figure 5d** Complex cysts are cysts with irregular features on CT. Some complex cysts are malignant.

or metastasis must grow to at least 5–10 mm before it will show up on a CT scan. Furthermore, small lymph nodes are often benign and a CT scan cannot differentiate this. One other important consideration is that intravenous contrast cannot be given to patients with poor kidney function because it can cause further damage to the kidneys. In these patients an MRI is usually the test of choice. Finally, for patients with complex cases of kidney cancer, CT scans must occasionally be combined with other radiographic tests to complete the evaluation.

Patient—Dennis W.:

*They were requiring me to have CT scans frequently. I expressed concern to my nurse and doctor that having only one kidney and having contrast run through my only existing kidney did not seem safe to me. After deliberation, they agreed to do the CTs less often, as long as there had been no significant change in my condition. By having this dialogue with my doctor and nurse, I had some productive input into my treatment.*

## 29. What is an MRI scan?

**Magnetic resonance imaging (MRI)**

A patient is placed in a magnetic field and radiofrequency signals are transmitted and received by surrounding coils. A computer processes the information and constructs cross-sectional images which provide detailed information on soft tissues.

In some ways **MRI** (known as **magnetic resonance imaging**) scans are even more powerful than CT scans. For this study the patient is brought through a scanner that detects magnetic signals from the atoms in each cell of the body and all of the information is stored on a computer (**Figure 6a**). Similar to CT, this information can then be displayed as "slices of the body" allowing us to visualize the internal anatomy.

One special advantage of MRI is that it is very strong at visualizing blood flow and for detecting tumors that are extending into veins. All malignant tumors have the potential to microscopically invade veins or capillaries. In fact, this is how they get into the bloodstream and metastasize to distant parts of the body. But kidney cancer is unusual in that it will often grow right into the renal vein (the main vein coming out of the kidney) and then into the inferior vena cava (the main vein going into the heart and the largest vein in the body). Occasionally it will grow right into the heart. This is known as a tumor thrombus (**Figure 6b**). Fortunately, most of these tumor thrombi can be removed surgically and a cure is still possible in many of these patients. When a tumor thrombus is suspected, an MRI is often the test of choice.

MRI is very good at showing local invasion of the cancer and beyond this can do almost all the things

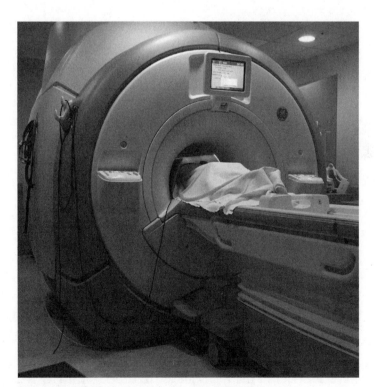

**Figure 6a** Magnetic resonance imaging (MRI) scanner.

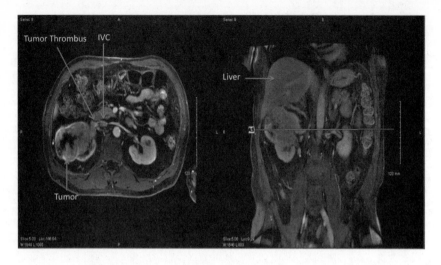

**Figure 6b** MRI image of renal cell carcinoma with tumor thrombus extending into the renal vein and inferior vena cava.

that a high-quality CT scan can do, as described in the previous section (**Figure 7**). MRI is the test of choice for patients with poor kidney function because it does not require intravenous contrast administration, which can cause further damage to the kidneys. MRI without contrast can often provide sufficient details about the kidney cancer, and when contrast is needed, different agents that are safe for the kidneys are used during MRI.

However, MRI does have some clear limitations. Some patients feel very claustrophobic and cannot tolerate MRI testing. Although these patients would prefer to have an "open" MRI, which is less claustrophobic, the images obtained are often suboptimal and this should be discouraged whenever possible. In addition, morbidly obese patients will often not "fit" into the scanners and patients with pacemakers or other metal objects cannot have an MRI in many instances. In summary, MRI is a

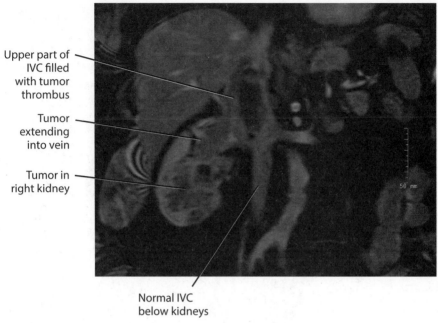

Upper part of
IVC filled
with tumor
thrombus

Tumor
extending
into vein

Tumor in
right kidney

50 mm

Normal IVC
below kidneys

**Figure 7** MRI image of renal cell carcinoma in right kidney.

very powerful test; however, it is very expensive and not required in most patients. It is best used selectively for patients with poor kidney function or when there is a suspicion of locally invasive cancer or venous tumor thrombus.

## 30. What is a bone scan?

A bone scan is used to look for bone metastasis, or spread of the cancer into the bones. For this test the patient is given a small intravenous dose of a radioisotope that tends to accumulate in inflamed or malignant areas of the bones. Later in the day the patient is scanned and the entire skeleton is visualized. Areas that light up are then evaluated to see what they may represent. Certain patterns are characteristic (**Figure 8a** and **Figure 8b**). Increased activity in the joints typically reflects arthritis.

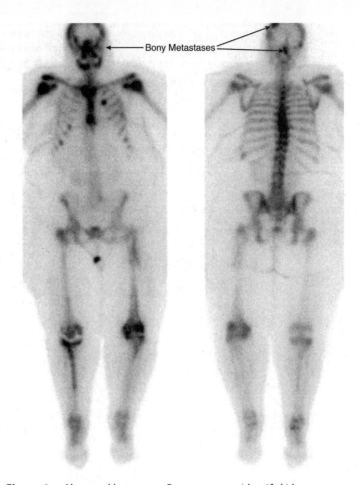

**Figure 8a** Abnormal bone scan. Bone scans can identify kidney cancer metastases to the bone because the uptake pattern is asymmetric, in this case within the skull. Metastases light up on this scan because they lead to inflammation within the bone. Radiologists can usually differentiate these abnormal findings from a normal bone scan, which has a symmetric pattern and only minimal uptake in the joints.

Another classic pattern is to see two or three adjacent ribs in a former football player light up signifying broken ribs from prior trauma. Other suspicious areas often require CT, MRI, and/or biopsy to see if they represent a metastasis of cancer. Most patients with kidney cancer do not need a bone scan. However, those with certain abnormal

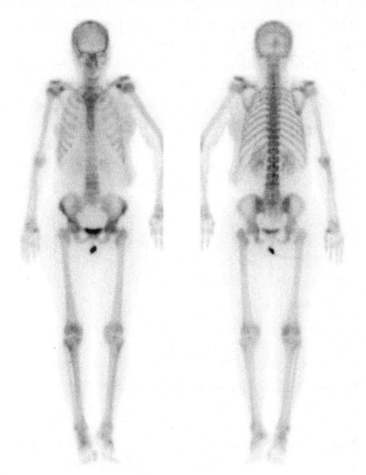

**Figure 8b** Normal bone scan from a patient with kidney cancer.

blood tests that reflect increased activity in the bones (alkaline phosphatase) and those with focal bone pain or a marked decline in their general condition due to fatigue or poor appetite should be considered for bone scan.

Many cancer patients worry about bone metastasis because they are elderly and have aches and pains from arthritis or slipped discs or other benign conditions. But cancer pain is usually distinctive and easy to differentiate from benign causes. One good rule of thumb is that cancer pain is typically relatively severe (difficult to relieve with pain medications), progressive (it gradually gets worse with time), often relentless, and not very dependent on position or activity level. This can be contrasted with arthritis, which can typically be relieved with aspirin-type medications, with changes in positioning, or with rest. Arthritis pain is also often directly related to certain activities, while cancer pain is not.

## 31. Is there a blood test for kidney cancer?

For some cancers, such as prostate cancer, specific blood tests will let us know if a patient is at risk. An elevated PSA (prostate-specific antigen) blood test suggests that the patient may have prostate cancer, and a biopsy can be considered to sort this out. For patients with prostate cancer, the PSA test can be used after treatment to monitor the activity of the cancer and to determine if it is still in remission. The PSA blood test is now considered the best such test in modern oncology.

Many patients ask whether there is a similar blood test for kidney cancer. Unfortunately, the answer is *no*. As of this point in time we still have no blood test for kidney cancer and this is true for most of the other cancers in the human body. Nevertheless, this is a very active area of research and new molecular technologies (proteomics and gene array analysis) hold great promise for identifying such a test in the future.

*Many benign kidney tumors, such as oncocytomas, look very much like kidney cancer under the microscope.*

## 32. Are there benign kidney tumors?

Patients often wonder: Could my tumor be benign? There are many benign kidney tumors, but most are uncommon and difficult to differentiate from kidney cancer prior to removal. **Table 5** lists some of the more important benign kidney tumors and their distinguishing characteristics. Some of these can be diagnosed by their appearance on X-rays.

- *Angiomyolipoma*, which has fat intermixed with the tumor, in most cases can be diagnosed by its appearance on CT.

- *Simple cysts*, which are water-filled cavities with thin walls, are very common and present distinctive findings on ultrasonography, CT, or MRI.

- *Minimally complex cysts*, which are fluid-filled cavities with thin septations or minimal calcification, or certain blood-filled cysts as long as they are otherwise benign appearing. These lesions are best characterized on CT scan or MRI—the risk of cancer is low (< 5%).

Most of the remaining benign renal tumors are difficult to differentiate from kidney cancer, although they can be suspected in certain populations. In general, benign renal tumors are more common in women, particularly young or middle-aged women. However, even in this population, the majority of solid, enhancing kidney tumors end up being malignant so most patients are best treated surgically. In this setting a partial nephrectomy should be considered, because we would prefer not to lose the entire kidney for a tumor that might end up being benign.

## 33. Will a biopsy help sort this out?

"Given that there are benign kidney tumors, shouldn't we do a biopsy to learn whether my tumor is benign or malignant?" This is the natural question that patients often ask. But there are problems with biopsies of kidney tumors. It is not like a lump in the breast where a biopsy can tell us in

**Table 5**  Benign Kidney Tumors

| Tumor Type | X-Ray Can Distinguish from Kidney Cancer | Distinguishing Characteristics |
|---|---|---|
| Angiomyolipoma | Yes | Contains fat intermixed with the tumor<br><br>Can bleed, so often treated if larger than 4cm |
| Oncocytoma | No | Particularly difficult to differentiate from kidney cancer based on X-rays or even with biopsy |
| Simple cyst | Yes | Very common; over half of population > 50 years of age has 1 or more kidney cyst |
| Minimally complex cyst | Yes | Risk of cancer is low, most patients are just observed |
| Cystic Nephroma | No | Most often seen in middle-aged women<br><br>Difficult to differentiate from cystic kidney cancer |
| Mixed Epithelial and Stromal Tumor of the Kidney (MESTK) | No | Most often seen in middle-aged women<br><br>Often associated with hormonal treatments |
| Metanephric Adenoma | No | More common in women |

a reliable manner whether it is benign or malignant, and we can make important decisions based on this.

Biopsies of kidney tumors are not perfectly accurate—they can suggest a tumor is benign when it is not, or vice versa, so they are difficult to trust. Part of the problem is that many of the benign kidney tumors, such as oncocytomas, look very much like kidney cancer under the microscope. So this is a very difficult call for the pathologist when they are given only a small biopsy. This is often referred to as "sampling error," since the pathologist can only evaluate a "sample" rather than the whole tumor. In fact it can be misleading and most of the time the final decision of benign versus malignant cannot be made until the entire tumor is removed. At best, an informative result can be obtained 80–90% of the time with biopsy, leaving 10–20% of patients with incomplete information and the potential for bleeding or other difficulties.

So if the X-rays suggest that a tumor is likely malignant the patient is usually treated for presumed malignancy, but must be aware that there is a chance that the final pathology may end up showing a benign tumor. Another way of putting this is that, for most patients, the biopsy is no more accurate than X-rays, so we elect to treat based upon the X-ray findings. However, there are some special circumstances where a biopsy can be useful:

- Patients with a history of another cancer, such as lung cancer. In this setting the biopsy is performed to learn whether the kidney tumor is a metastasis from the other cancer. If so, the treatment is chemotherapy for lung cancer rather than surgery for kidney cancer.

- Patients with enlarged lymph nodes in a pattern that suggests lymphoma. If the biopsy shows lymphoma rather than kidney cancer, the main treatment is chemotherapy rather than surgery.

- Patients with a fever and urinary tract infection. In certain settings the "tumor" may actually be an abscess (infected cavity). If the biopsy shows this, the treatment is antibiotics rather than surgery.

- Some patients with advanced kidney cancer where a biopsy will tell us the type of kidney cancer and help guide therapy.
- Patients in whom the recommended treatment would change significantly based on the results of a biopsy, such as a patient with increased surgical risk that would be managed with surveillance unless a particularly aggressive cancer were diagnosed at biopsy.
- Patients should undergo biopsy prior to, or at the time of, thermal ablation of a renal tumor.

It is important to emphasize that these situations are in the minority—many patients do not benefit from a biopsy and should not be exposed to the risk that this procedure can carry. Some centers are now performing more biopsies to learn more about the procedure and to improve it, and this is a very reasonable approach. In the future, biopsy will likely be performed more often, and when combined with molecular testing, there is a vision that it will provide more accurate information and will be very helpful for guiding patient management.

# PART FOUR

# Staging of Renal Cell Carcinoma

How is kidney cancer staged?

What does tumor grade mean?

What is a tumor thrombus?

*More*\*...

*Words that may not be familiar to you are included in the glossary. We have highlighted them in **bold** when they are first used in this book.

## 34. How is kidney cancer staged?

By staging your cancer, your doctor is trying to assess whether your kidney cancer is confined to the kidney and, if not, to what extent it has moved outside of your kidney. Staging is one of the most important prognostic or predictive factors in kidney cancer.

There are two staging procedures for all cancers. The first is called clinical staging while the second is pathological staging. Clinical staging is based on radiographic findings (chest X-ray, CT scan, MRIs, bone scans, etc). While evaluating the CT or MRI, your doctor is looking for any evidence of cancer spread outside the kidney such as into the nearby fat, muscle, lymph nodes, adrenal glands, or other organs (**Figure 9**). Additional testing sometimes includes a bone scan and imaging of the brain. In the absence of suspicious bony or neurological symptoms, most patients do not need these additional tests—studies have shown them to be negative in the overwhelming majority of asymptomatic patients.

Cancer stages are designated using the TNM system which is updated periodically by the American Joint Commission on Cancer (AJCC). T refers to local tumor extent, N refers to lymph nodes, and M refers to any distant metastases (cancer outside the kidney or lymph nodes). Your doctor will then assign you a TNM stage and based on this an overall stage (I–IV). Radiology tests are limited in their ability to detect microscopic disease that has escaped the kidney. In other words, even though the results of your clinical staging may be encouraging, the pathological staging is even more important.

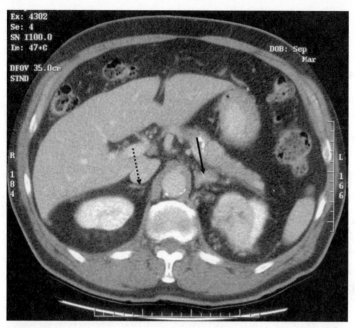

**Figure 9a** Renal cell carcinoma can metastasize to the adrenal gland which lies next to the kidney. Note that the normal gland (dotted line on patient's right) is smaller than the gland containing cancer (solid line on patient's left).

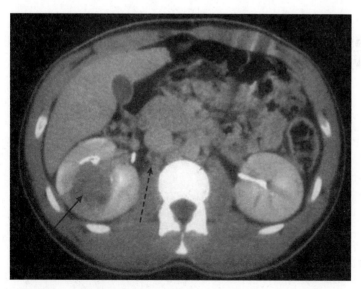

**Figure 9b** A kidney tumor (solid line) can also spread to lymph nodes near the kidney (dotted line).

The pathological staging is assigned by your doctor after you have had surgery and the pathologist can look microscopically to determine exactly how advanced the cancer has become. The pathologist looks specifically to see if there is microscopic disease in the nearby fat, muscle, adrenal gland, lymph nodes, and/or kidney veins based on a detailed study of the surgical specimen (**Figure 10**). It is important to understand that while the clinical and pathological stages often agree, there are times where they do not. In these circumstances, the pathological stage is more important. It is also possible that the pathological stage may underestimate the microscopic extent of your kidney cancer. In other words, microscopic cells may have escaped your kidney but eluded all means of detection. In these cases, there are no tests that can detect residual microscopic cells. Unfortunately, positron emission tomography (PET) scans are *not* accurate for staging kidney cancer in most circumstances. New radiology studies, including an antibody called G250, are being tested; however, these tests are still experimental and unproven.

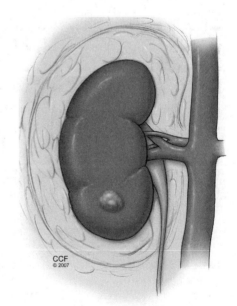

### Figure 10a

Staging of renal cell carcinoma. Tumor (T) stage incorporates the size and invasiveness of the tumor. The N and M stage are determined by the presence or absence of lymph node and distant metastases. T1a (10a) and T1b (10b) tumors are confined to the kidney. Tumors < 4 cm are classified as T1a and 4–7 cm as T1b.

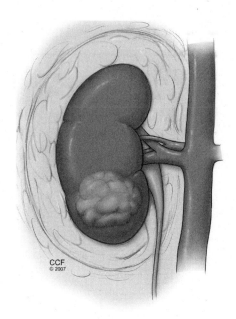

### Figure 10b

T1b tumor

Reprinted with permission, Cleveland Clinic Center for Medical Art & Photography © 2007–2014. All Rights Reserved.

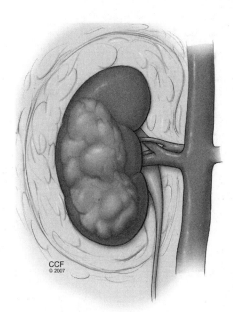

**Figure 10c** T2 tumors are > 7cm and confined to the kidney. T2a and T2b tumors are confined to the kidney and between 7 and 10 cm and larger than 10 cm, respectively.

Reprinted with permission, Cleveland Clinic Center for Medical Art & Photography © 2007–2014. All Rights Reserved.

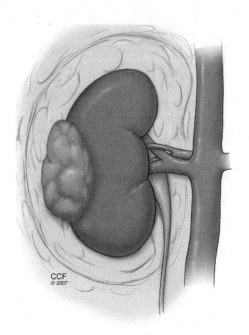

### Figure 10d

T3a tumors invade the fat around or in the center or the kidney OR the renal vein or its branches. It does not involve any areas beyond its containing tissues (Gerota's fascia).

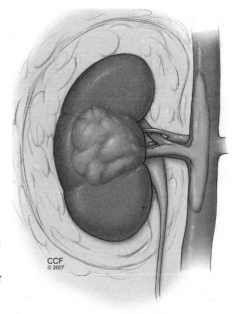

### Figure 10e

T3b tumors extend into the vena cava below the diaphragm.

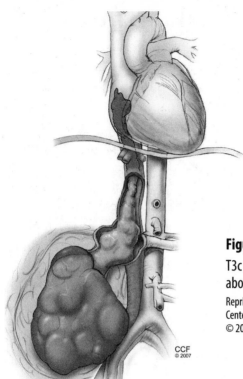

**Figure 10f**

T3c tumors extend into vena cava above diaphragm.

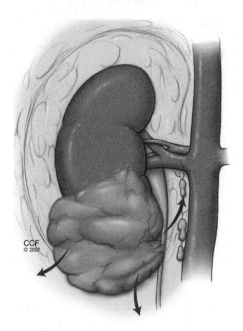

**Figure 10g**

T4 tumors extend into nearby organs such as the liver, the bowel, or the adrenal gland.

## 35. What does tumor grade mean?

All tumors are given a tumor grade. This refers to how aggressive the cells appear when examined under the microscope. Tumor grade cannot be determined by any radiology test. Only the pathologist can determine the tumor grade. What the pathologist looks for is how similar the kidney cancer cells are to normal, noncancerous kidney cells. The more the kidney cancer looks like a noncancerous normal kidney, the lower the tumor grade and the better the prognosis. The less the kidney cancer looks like noncancerous normal kidney, the higher the tumor grade. High-grade cancer cells are angry looking and are associated with a worse prognosis.

Your tumor may be graded in different ways, depending on the pathologist and the type of kidney tumor. The most common grading system is based on the appearance of the nucleus of the kidney cancer cell, where the chromosomes reside (**Figure 11**). In clear cell renal cell carcinoma (RCC) this is the Fuhrman system and is on a scale of 1 to 4. Fuhrman grade 1 and 2 are "low grade" and Fuhrman grade 3 and 4 tumors are "high grade." If you do not have a clear cell RCC, the pathologist may not give a Fuhrman grade. For other types of kidney cancer including papillary or chromophobe RCC, the pathologist may simply refer to the tumor as Type 1/low grade or Type 2/high grade. There is no single parameter that determines your prognosis. While higher grades predict potentially more aggressive tumors, these values must be interpreted in the context of other factors. In practice, tumor grade and stage are combined with several other factors to determine your prognosis.

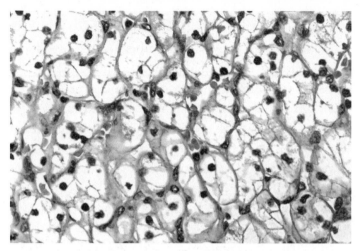

**Figure 11a** The histologic appearance of renal cell carcinoma can vary significantly under the microscope. Low-grade clear cell renal cell carcinoma is made up of cells that all look similar, are of normal size, and contain normal nuclei.

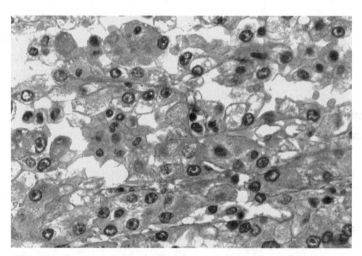

**Figure 11b** In contrast, a high-grade tumor contains bizarre-appearing cells with abnormal nuclei. The nuclear grade of RCC (grade 1–4) provides information about the aggressiveness of the tumor, with higher grade predicting more aggressive clinical behavior.

## 36. What is a tumor thrombus?

The kidneys are very efficient filters of the blood and are therefore very vascular. They filter more than 1 liter of blood per minute and have a complex vascular network. As kidney cancers progress they may extend into nearby small veins that drain blood out of the kidney. This causes the body's natural defenses to attack the tumor cells. During this process, platelets and other immune cells clump together with tumor cells and may form a blood clot. This is called a tumor thrombus.

While a tumor thrombus starts in the smallest of blood vessels it can progress into larger kidney veins and out the main kidney vein (renal vein thrombus). From there, the thrombus can extend up the inferior vena cava (**Figure 12**), the largest vein in the body. The inferior vena cava is responsible for returning all the blood from below the diaphragm back to the heart. The tumor thrombus can then extend into nearby liver veins or even into the right side of the heart. Surgery to remove the tumor thrombus can be very complex depending on its level.

If the thrombus is within the renal vein or just barely entering the inferior vena cava, it is a level 1 thrombus. If it extends into the vena cava below the liver veins it is a level 2 thrombus and requires more surgical expertise. Once it is above the liver veins (level 3) or into the heart (level 4), you may require heart bypass or sophisticated venous bypass. These operations are very challenging and typically require collaboration between your urologist and a heart or vascular surgeon to safely remove the thrombus.

**Bland thrombus**

A blood clot inside of a vein. This is in contrast to the growth of tumor cells within the vein, that can occur in kidney cancer patients.

Not all tumor thrombi have active cancer cells within them. Some thrombi, called **bland thrombi**, have no

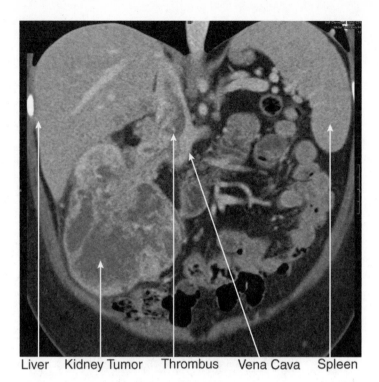

Liver   Kidney Tumor   Thrombus   Vena Cava   Spleen

**Figure 12a** CT image of renal cell carcinoma with tumor thrombus within the renal vein and inferior vena cava.

cancer cells inside them, although they are usually associated with other areas of malignant tumor thrombus. Usually a bland thrombus is found in the vena cava below the kidney veins.

It is important for you to know what level your thrombus has reached because this impacts the extent and risk of surgery. If the thrombus is not removed, there is a risk for an embolism of the thrombus, usually to the lungs, which can be fatal. The surgery and postoperative care are much more involved in patients with tumor thrombus. All patients with a tumor thrombus are considered at least stage III.

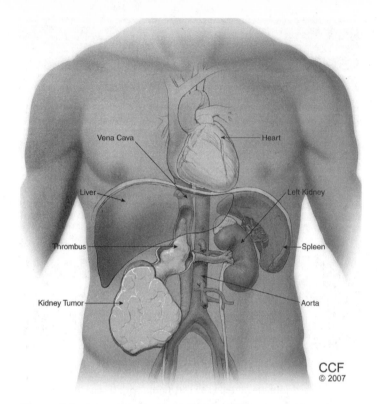

**Figure 12b** Schematic demonstrating the kidney tumor, thrombus, and nearby structures present on the corresponding CT image.

## 37. What is a lymph node? How are the lymph nodes involved in kidney cancer?

As the blood circulates through your blood vessels some of the fluid inevitably seeps out. A nice analogy is to look at a pipe of cold water on a hot day. Some of the fluid is condensed on the outside of the pipe. If there were no way to reclaim the fluid that shifted out of the vessels or out of the cells, we would become dehydrated very quickly. To prevent this, the body has developed an elaborate series of channels (lymphatics) and filters (lymph nodes) to reclaim this fluid.

Lymph nodes are filters that recycle this fluid back into the bloodstream. They are an important point where the immune system can trap foreign cells or cancer cells and begin to fight the cancer. If cancer cells escape the organ where they began, they can be trapped in lymph nodes. There are lymph nodes associated with all the organs in the body, and the first lymph nodes to be involved are typically those that are right near the organ with the cancer. For the kidney, the commonly involved lymph nodes lie adjacent to the kidney next to the aorta and inferior vena cava (**Figure 13**). If these lymph nodes are enlarged on CT or MRI, they should be removed with your kidney at the time of surgery. Patients with lymph node involvement from kidney cancer have stage III or IV disease depending on the extent of the tumor (T stage) and the presence or absence of metastases (M stage). In general, these patients are at a higher risk of recurrence. Anytime the cancer is aggressive enough to get into the lymph nodes, it is considered a higher risk cancer.

## 38. Where does kidney cancer spread to?

Most kidney cancers have potential to spread to other parts of the body. The risk of this depends on a number of factors as discussed above. When doctors think of spread from kidney cancer they consider two types or categories of spread: local spread and distant spread (metastases). Local spread from kidney cancer starts with invasion of nearby structures. The kidney has a capsule that holds it together. Kidney cancer cells can escape through this capsule into nearby fat or the adrenal gland sitting above the kidney. If very aggressive, it can invade nearby muscles or adjacent organs (liver, pancreas, intestines, or diaphragm). Additionally, the cancer can spread outside the kidney via either lymphatic or

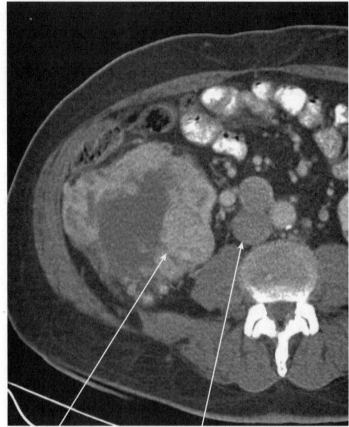

Kidney Tumor    Enlarged Lymph Node

**Figure 13** Lymph node metastasis. Kidney cancer can spread into the nearby lymph nodes, which become enlarged. Normally, lymph nodes are not well identified on CT scan, but enlarged lymph nodes can be quite pronounced.

blood vessels. When this occurs, the cancer can get into the lymph nodes or into the main bloodstream allowing it to spread throughout the body. The most common sites of distant spread (metastasis) are the lungs, liver, bones, and brain (**Table 6**; **Figure 14**); kidney cancer can also occasionally spread to unusual locations such as the skin, eyes, mouth, and gallbladder. Fortunately, metastases to these locations are rare.

**Table 6** Site of Metastases, Relative Incidence, and Median Time to Recur

| Site of Recurrence | Incidence | Median Time to Recur (Years) |
|---|---|---|
| Lung | 38% | 1.6 |
| Bone | 18% | 1.5 |
| Liver | 13% | 1.7 |
| Local (includes adrenal) | 10% | 1.7 |
| CNS (brain and spinal cord) | 8% | 2.5 |

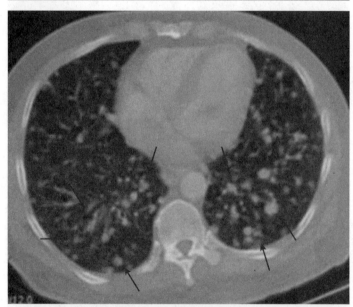

**Figure 14a**

Kidney cancer metastasis to lung.

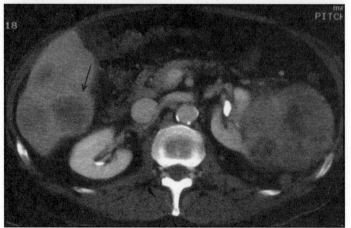

**Figure 14b**

Kidney cancer metastasis to liver.

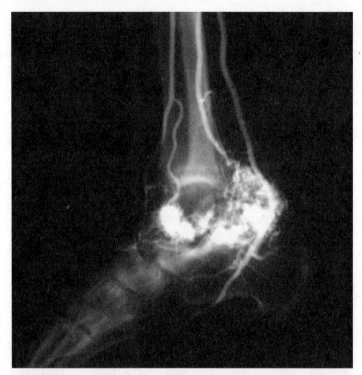

**Figure 14c**
Kidney cancer metastasis to bone.

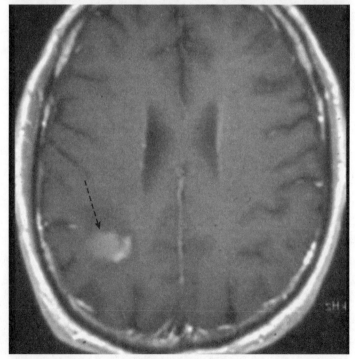

**Figure 14d**
Kidney cancer metastasis to brain.

## 39. What symptoms do metastases cause?

Symptoms from kidney cancer can be due to local disease or metastases. The most common local symptom is hematuria (microscopic or visible blood in the urine). Other local symptoms are less specific, including pain or symptoms caused by the mass pressing on nearby organs or nerves. Most patients with advanced RCC (50–80%) are asymptomatic with metastases picked up incidentally by CT scan, MRI, or X-ray. This is unfortunate because having symptoms might have caused the cancer to be discovered sooner. When symptoms do occur, the nature of these symptoms depends on the location of the metastases, the size of the metastases, and their effects on nearby organs.

Many symptoms are nonspecific including fever, fatigue, poor appetite, and weight loss. Metastatic kidney cancer can cause symptoms related to the organ that is involved, such as cough or blood in the sputum (lung), itching and jaundice (liver), pain in the bones, neurological signs (brain or spinal cord), and many other uncommon symptoms depending on location. Many patients with kidney cancer attribute any or all symptoms they experience to their fear that their kidney cancer has recurred. In fact, if you are being followed regularly and if your scans are negative, it is unlikely that your symptoms are due to recurrent or advanced kidney cancer.

## 40. What is a paraneoplastic syndrome?

Hormones are substances, usually proteins, that are released into the bloodstream to regulate our bodily functions. A good example is insulin, which is released by the pancreas and controls our blood sugar levels. Normal kidney cells make certain hormones that regulate our

**Erythropoietin**

A hormone that stimulates production of red blood cells and hemoglobin in the bone marrow. This hormone is overproduced by some kidney tumors leading to high red blood cell counts, the opposite of anemia.

**Hemoglobin**

The oxygen-carrying component in red blood cells that gives them their red color and serves to bring oxygen to the tissues.

**Hematocrit**

Blood test that measures the thickness of the blood, which is a reflection of its oxygen-carrying capacity. The hematocrit value is the ratio of the volume occupied by packed red blood cells to the volume of the whole blood.

**Viscosity**

The resistance of a substance to flow.

**Parathormone**

A hormone synthesized and released into the bloodstream by the parathyroid glands; regulates phosphorus and calcium in the body and functions in neuromuscular excitation and blood clotting.

blood pressure and blood counts. Occasionally kidney cancer cells will become dysregulated and overproduce these hormones or other hormones that are normally made by other organ systems. This can cause symptoms depending on which hormone is overproduced (**Table 7**). This is called a paraneoplastic syndrome. For example, normal kidney cells are responsible for stimulating the bone marrow to produce red blood cells by manufacturing **erythropoietin**. If a kidney tumor overproduces erythropoietin, this can cause a patient's **hemoglobin** and **hematocrit** levels to rise, which may cause symptoms related to increased blood **viscosity** such as the clogging of small arteries.

Another example of a paraneoplastic syndrome is the overproduction of renin, which normal kidney cells make to control our blood pressure. If renin is overproduced by the tumor, this may lead to high blood pressure that can be dangerous if extreme. If **parathormone** is overproduced, the patient may develop signs of high calcium levels such as muscle or joint pains or neurologic symptoms.

**Table 7** Paraneoplastic Syndromes Associated with RCC

| Finding | Incidence |
| --- | --- |
| Cachexia (weight loss)/fever | 20–33% |
| High blood pressure | 25% |
| High calcium | 20% |
| Low blood counts (anemia) | 20–40% |
| Diabetes (hyperglycemia) | 10–20% |
| Liver dysfunction (Stauffer's syndrome) | 3–20% |
| High blood counts (erythrocytosis) | 1–8% |
| Amyloidosis | 3–5% |

Kidney cancer is notorious for causing paraneoplastic syndromes—of all the human cancers it is the one that is associated with the most divergent array of such syndromes. This is one of the major challenges that some kidney cancer patients face, since these syndromes can be symptomatic and occasionally disabling.

Diagnosis of a paraneoplastic syndrome requires a high index of suspicion and clinical awareness on the part of the physician. Diagnosis is usually made by the combination of symptoms in conjunction with abnormal lab values. Often, the paraneoplastic symptoms will lessen after removal of a localized tumor. In cases of metastatic kidney cancer, treatment is directed at killing the cancer cells or simply treating a specific problem such as high serum calcium.

## 41. What causes weight loss or fatigue?

Many patients with kidney cancer experience symptoms affecting their overall sense of well being including unexplained weight loss and fatigue. There is rarely a single cause for these "constitutional symptoms" but rather multiple contributing factors including physical and emotional stress, poor sleeping habits, and in some cases overproduction of inflammatory hormones (cytokines) as part of a paraneoplastic syndrome. During the evaluation and treatment of kidney cancer, your mind and body are going through much turmoil. Many patients find relaxation or meditation techniques essential to maintaining a positive outlook. Moreover, immediately after surgery or during systemic therapy for kidney cancer, your body requires additional calories to rebuild. It is important that you work with your family, your doctor, and a nutritionist if necessary to maintain your weight and combat excess weight loss.

Occasionally following surgery or during systemic therapies, excess fatigue can also be a sign of anemia. In this case, your doctor may recommend blood transfusions or more rarely erythropoietin. There are several formulations of injectable erythropoietin, so you will have to check with your doctor.

Patient—Dennis W.:

*At one point during my treatment, I had lost about 35 pounds, was very weak, and my stomach was distended. I had several liters of fluid drawn from my abdomen and had a hard time breathing and eating. My martial arts teacher started doing breathing exercises with me and taught me several advanced methods to use on my own to help strengthen my lungs and restore my energy. There is no doubt in my mind, this was significant in my recovery. I encourage anyone who has a similar condition to stay as active as you can, including mind, body, and spirit.*

Caregiver—Linda C.:

*Throughout Lori's treatment she lost more than 100 pounds. At 5'8" she was very self-conscious of this weight loss. She tried hard to gain weight, as she knew her body needed these calories. Because she did not like the nutritional drinks available in the stores, her oncologist suggested another brand. It had double the calories and Lori actually enjoyed the taste. We froze the drink and whole milk in ice cube trays and made fruit smoothies. This gave the drinks more nutrition and also added calories.*

*Many times your loved one will not feel like eating. Lori said seeing a plate full of food was overwhelming many times and almost made her sick to look at it. Sometimes she chose not to come to the table at meal time. If he/she is in bed, like Lori was for many meals, it is important to make his/her tray look appealing. I would sometimes use her pretty dishes, and sometimes put a flower on the tray. It is also more enjoyable for the patient if he/she has someone eat with him/her—(it's no fun eating alone). She always ate better if someone ate with her.*

*Lori had to have many blood transfusions. I cannot stress the importance of donating blood to everyone who can donate! You can save a life by this small gesture. When you think of what your loved one is going through—the time involved and the bit of discomfort is NOTHING to what he/she is going through! Please give blood!*

## 42. Do patients die from kidney cancer?

First, the majority of patients with kidney cancer do not die of their disease. Since kidney cancer is more common in elderly patients, often there are other medical conditions that have a higher likelihood of causing a patient's demise. Moreover, kidney cancer can act very differently among patients.

Unfortunately, each year in the United States approximately 13,000 people will die from kidney cancer. Many of these patients will have advanced or aggressive disease at the time of their diagnosis. There is often no single precipitating event that causes death in a patient with kidney cancer. Since the disease can involve many different organs, death from advanced disease is usually due to a combination of medical issues causing gradual weight loss and failure to thrive. Patients may become very fatigued, develop a poor appetite, or become intolerant of food and liquids. In some instances, patients with advanced disease may develop an acute medical event such as a blood clot or embolism to the lung, seizures, or a life-threatening infection.

Fortunately, the majority of patients who die of kidney cancer do not experience pain or severe discomfort. In most hospitals and cancer centers, patients and families are encouraged to speak with each other and are given multiple resources to deal with end-of-life issues and concerns. Death with dignity is a frequently achieved goal in patients with terminal kidney cancer.

Caregiver—Linda C.:

*Yes, patients die from kidney cancer! My daughter Lori was diagnosed at the age of 32. She fought as hard as she could so she could raise her four children, but was unable to find a treatment that would stop this disease. She passed away at the age of 34, leaving children ages 2, 3, 11, and 17. We must stop this disease from taking other children's mothers!*

# PART FIVE

# *Treatment: Localized Disease*

How is kidney cancer treated?

What are the treatment options for localized (Stage I–II) kidney tumors?

What is the prognosis for patients with localized kidney tumors?

*More*\*...

## 43. How is kidney cancer treated?

Surgery is the primary treatment for kidney cancer, particularly for patients with localized disease. Surgery is curative in the majority of such patients and offers the best chance for long-term survival. Most treatments therefore begin with removal of the kidney in full or part. Surgical options include radical nephrectomy (total removal), partial nephrectomy, and/or tumor destruction (ablation). Each of these procedures can be done via an open approach (a standard incision), laparoscopically or robotically (via telescopes and instruments inserted into ports—small incisions—placed through the body wall), and in some cases **percutaneously** (under CT, MRI, or US [ultrasound] guidance).

In patients with more advanced disease, treatment is often multimodal, meaning that, in addition to surgery, a systemic treatment is given to try to reduce the risk of recurrence or to combat any known or hidden disease outside the kidney. In these cases, surgery is often performed first, followed by systemic therapies. In some instances, physicians may choose to treat a patient with systemic therapies first and operate on a patient after an initial course of medical therapy. With this approach, the effect of the systemic therapy can be observed prior to a major operation; in some cases, treatment can downsize the tumor and make it much easier to remove surgically. Because this treatment strategy (known as **neoadjuvant therapy**) has not yet been proven, it is often best to do it as part of a clinical trial. An overview of the treatments for kidney cancer is provided in Table 4 in **Part Two**.

Radiation therapy is rarely used as a treatment for patients with kidney cancer except in patients with metastases to

**Percutaneous**

With regards to kidney cancer, refers to treatments performed by inserting a needle through the skin without further need for incisions.

**Neoadjuvant therapy**

Treatment given as a first step to shrink a tumor before the main treatment, which is usually surgery, is given. Examples of neoadjuvant therapy include chemotherapy, radiation therapy, and hormone therapy. It is a type of induction therapy.

the bone, brain, or spinal cord. In these instances, radiation therapy can reduce the local pressure of the tumor on normal structures. In this setting radiation therapy can relieve acute symptoms such as disabling pain, but it tends not to be curative. Depending on many factors including a patient's age, other medical problems, the size of the tumor, the presence of associated symptoms, and the patient's wishes, treatment for early kidney cancers may sometimes be deferred or delayed.

Recent studies suggest that in selected, usually elderly, patients with competing health risks and stage I kidney cancers < 4 cm, the growth rate of the tumor may be either very slow or the tumor may not grow at all. In these instances, the physician and patient together may choose a course of **active surveillance** and follow the tumor's radiographic size and appearance. Although this is not considered an active form of treatment, it underscores the point that in some patients these tumors can be relatively slow growing and non-life-threatening. Younger and/or relatively healthy patients should consider a more proactive approach because there is a risk of cancer progression with surveillance alone.

**Active surveillance**
Active surveillance is also known as watchful waiting or observation and simply means that a physician and a patient work together to actively observe an identified renal mass. Radiographic tests such as a CT scan, MRI scan, or ultrasound are done at regular intervals to observe the mass.

## 44. What are the treatment options for localized (Stage I–II) kidney tumors?

Patients with stage I or II renal cell carcinoma (RCC) have disease confined to the kidney. The only difference between stage I and II RCC is the size of the tumor. Stage I kidney cancer is separated into stage I-a (< 4 cm) and I-b (4–7 cm) while stage II kidney cancer is also separated into II-a (7–10 cm) and II-b (> 7 cm). All are confined to the kidney.

*Surgery is the primary treatment for kidney cancer, particularly for patients with localized disease.*

Options for stage I or II RCC include:
- Partial nephrectomy
- Radical nephrectomy
- Tumor ablation
- Observation, also known as active surveillance

Treatment decisions depend on many factors including age; other medical problems; risks of anesthesia; the size, location, and invasiveness of the tumor; and a physician's training and experience performing these procedures. In general, for larger tumors (> 7 cm) or higher stage tumors, a complete removal of the kidney, or radical nephrectomy, is probably best if the other kidney is functioning normally. If removal of the kidney puts the patient at a high risk of needing dialysis all efforts should be made toward a partial nephrectomy to save as much kidney function as possible. Other general considerations for stages I and II kidney cancer include whether the tumor is central or involves the main blood vessels or drainage tubes of the kidney. It should be emphasized that current data suggest that partial removal and total removal of the kidney have equivalent rates of cure for most localized kidney cancers and the decision to pursue one over the other depends on many factors including the experience and expertise of the doctor you see.

**Tumor ablation**

Killing tumor cells directly using heat or cold or other types of energy. This is done laparoscpically or by percutaneous treatment.

**Tumor ablation** refers to destruction of the tumor and a portion of nearby normal kidney using one of two methods: extreme cooling/freezing (cryotherapy) or superheating (radiofrequency ablation) of the tumor. These two methods are best reserved for small (< 3 cm), peripheral tumors in patients who are poor surgical candidates due to advanced age or other medical problems. Tumor ablation can be done laparoscopically/robotically (see Question 50) or percutaneously, through the skin, again depending on the anatomy. In highly selected patients, active surveillance (observation) may be an option if the tumor is believed to be small and indolent (slow growing). This approach is best reserved for patients with small tumors and requires close radiographic surveillance to assess growth.

All treatment options have unique risks and benefits. The *general principles of surgical treatment for stage I and II kidney cancer* can be summarized as follows:

- Smaller lesions (< 7 cm) are best treated by partial nephrectomy.

- Ablation remains most appropriate in less aggressive tumors in elderly patients or patients with limited life expectancy.

- Large lesions (> 7 cm) are generally treated by radical nephrectomy unless there is a risk of dialysis (tumors in both kidneys, tumor in a solitary kidney, or impaired kidney function).

- For localized RCC, the risk of recurrence appears equally low following radical or partial nephrectomy. The benefit of partial nephrectomy is that it spares normal kidney and best preserves overall function.

- Most radical nephrectomies can be performed laparoscopically in experienced hands.

- Many partial nephrectomies can be approached laparoscopically or robotically.

- The choice of which approach is best for you depends very much on your doctor's experience and your willingness to accept the possible risks associated with that approach.

The *general principles of stage III and IV kidney cancer* can be summarized as follows:

- Surgery is recommended to remove the primary tumor and all locally enlarged lymph nodes.

- All renal vein or vena caval thrombus should be removed unless it would be unsafe to do so—but here too this requires the judgment of an experienced kidney cancer surgeon as it is uncommon and not recommended to leave thrombus in place with the surgery.

- Depending on the location, timing, and number of metastases, it may be recommended that an aggressive surgical approach be taken to remove these in addition to the cancerous kidney.

- High-risk patients rendered surgically free of disease may be offered **adjuvant treatment**, usually in a clinical trial.

- Most patients with persistent or recurrent disease after surgery require systemic therapy.

- Multimodal therapy (surgery plus systemic therapy) is typically prioritized for patients with advanced kidney cancer. This requires that you have at least two kidney cancer experts on your team—a surgeon (urologic oncologist) and a medical oncologist.

Since many surgical options are available to patients with stage I and II kidney cancer, you may hear differences in opinion from the doctors you see. Each doctor's recommendation is likely to be affected by his training and comfort level with a given approach. Many doctors may not have trained to perform sophisticated kidney preservations (partial nephrectomy) or laparoscopic/robotic kidney surgery, and this can influence their advice.

**Adjuvant treatment**

Utilizing medications, radiation therapy, or other means of supplemental treatment following cancer surgery.

## 45. What is the prognosis for patients with localized kidney tumors?

More than half of all patients with kidney cancer present with stage I or II disease, with the tumor still confined to the kidney. In these patients, surgery is the main treatment option. Fortunately, surgery cures the majority of patients with localized disease. In patients with stage Ia disease, recurrence is uncommon (90–95% remain cancer free). In stage Ib disease, 80–90% remain cancer free, and for stage II about 75–80% remain cancer free.

What makes the risk of localized disease so low in some patients while higher in others? The most important prognostic factors other than stage are grade and type of kidney cancer.

Conventional (clear cell) kidney cancer tends to carry higher risk than papillary or chromophobe variants, and high grade always increases the risk of recurrence. Other factors that may predict recurrence include age, performance status (how debilitated a patient is as a result of the tumor), the presence of tumor-related symptoms, microscopic vein involvement, microscopic tumor necrosis (dead cancer cells within the tumor proper), and certain lab tests (platelet count, sedimentation rate, calcium levels, etc.).

Of all these factors, tumor stage is the most important, and patients with low-stage tumors that are still confined to the kidney tend to do well, although this is not uniformly true. Importantly there are statistical models that physicians can use to predict recurrence rates. These models require the physician to input your specific variables and from there they can calculate rates based on patients who have had similar risk

**Laparoscopic**

Pertaining to laparoscopy, such as laparoscopic surgery. A fiber optic camera and instrument, passed through a small incision in the abdominal wall and equipped with instruments with which to examine the abdominal cavity or perform surgery. Some laparoscopic surgeries are also performed with a robotic surgical system, and termed "robot-assisted laparoscopic" or "robotic" surgeries.

**Laparoscopy**

Use of small instruments and telescopes (cameras that look inside the body) to access various compartments of the body. Carbon dioxide gas is pumped into the body through small channels in order to create space between the abdominal wall and the intraabdominal organs facilitating the operation.

**Transperitoneal**

Through the peritoneum, the smooth membrane that lines the abdominal cavity.

profiles. These models are called nomograms. You can ask your physician what your nomogram results are postoperatively. The nomograms are also available at *www.cancernomograms.com*, which your physician can help you navigate.

## 46. What is a radical nephrectomy?

Radical nephrectomy refers to complete surgical removal of the kidney. In the classically described operation, a radical nephrectomy refers to removal of the kidney, all the surrounding fat, the adrenal glands, and nearby lymph nodes.

Over the course of the last 20–30 years, radical nephrectomy has become less "radical." Adrenalectomy is now routinely avoided unless there is a high suspicion for involvement at the time of surgery. Moreover, lymph nodes are often removed only if enlarged. Different surgical approaches include open and laparoscopic/robotic radical nephrectomy. An open approach describes an incision made in the body wall, typically along the flank, to remove the kidney. It usually does not require excision of any ribs or muscles. **Laparoscopic** approaches for radical nephrectomy include "pure" **laparoscopy**, via a **transperitoneal** or retroperitoneal technique, or a hand-assisted approach (see Question 50). Pure laparoscopic requires the most technical expertise and is the least invasive. The surgeon uses instruments inserted through ports, or tiny skin incisions, to disconnect and remove the kidney. In the hand-assisted approach the surgeon inserts a hand to assist in a laparoscopic removal of the kidney.

The transperitoneal approach involves approaching the kidney through the abdominal cavity. In the retroperitoneal approach, the kidney is accessed from the back, staying out of the abdominal cavity completely. Both approaches have advantages and disadvantages. Advantages of the retroperitoneal approach include avoiding sites of prior surgery and avoiding mobilization of the bowels. Your surgeon will determine which type of procedure is best for you based on your CT or MRI scans and other factors including his or her experience with these techniques.

During a laparoscopic radical nephrectomy, the kidney is entrapped in an internal bag and removed through a small incision. In the past, some surgeons would **morcellate** or fragment the kidney inside the body (in the entrapment bag) prior to removing it. Although fragmenting the kidney may be used when the kidney is removed for noncancerous conditions, this procedure is generally not performed during removal of kidney tumors because it may increase the risk of tumor spillage, which increases the risk of recurrence, and may also prevent accurate pathological assessment.

Over the last decade the laparoscopic approach has become standard for most radical nephrectomies. These approaches are less invasive and facilitate more rapid recovery and should be considered if possible. In general, the relative reasons NOT to perform a nephrectomy laparoscopically are few and include tumor thrombus, a very large tumor (> 10–15 cm), and/or bulky lymph node enlargement.

Finally, evidence suggests that radical nephrectomy may be "overtreatment" for many kidney cancers. Patients undergoing radical nephrectomy are at slightly higher risk for kidney failure because they are left with a solitary kidney. It is imperative that you ask your surgeon about kidney preservation (partial nephrectomy). If your

**Morcellate**

Because minimally-invasive, laparoscopic techniques use only small incisions, some surgeons have performed this technique to break larger specimens into smaller pieces so they can be removed without making a larger incision. This has not been done routinely for cancer specimens so that they can be examined as whole tumors by the pathologist after they have been removed.

tumor is less than 4–7 cm, you are probably a candidate for kidney sparing. Your surgeon's experience in performing the operation is of paramount importance.

## 47. What is a partial nephrectomy?

*Kidney preservation is an important goal during the treatment of RCC.*

Kidney preservation is an important goal during the treatment of RCC. Partial nephrectomy refers to removal of the tumorous portion and a small margin of normal kidney (**Figure 15**).

Partial nephrectomy is performed for absolute, relative, and elective indications (**Table 8**). Absolute indications include patients with a tumor in a solitary kidney or tumors in both kidneys. In these cases, radical

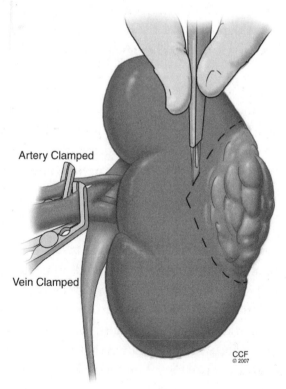

Artery Clamped

Vein Clamped

CCF
© 2007

**Figure 15a** Schematic of open partial nephrectomy. After taking fat off of the surface of the kidney, the arteries and veins to the kidney are clamped to block blood flow to the kidney temporarily.

Reprinted with permission, Cleveland Clinic Center for Medical Art & Photography © 2007–2014. All Rights Reserved.

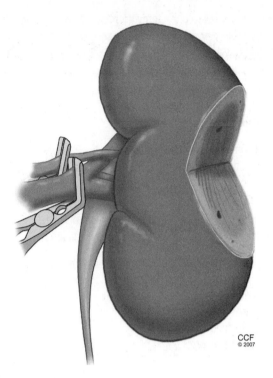

**Figure 15b**
The tumor is then excised sharply with a thin margin of normal tissue.

Reprinted with permission, Cleveland Clinic Center for Medical Art & Photography © 2007–2014. All Rights Reserved.

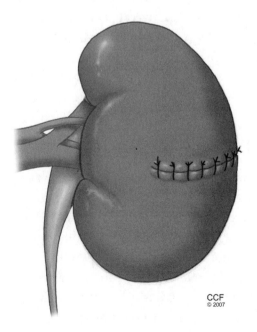

**Figure 15c** After removing the kidney tumor, reconstruction of the kidney is performed with sutures to close the capsule which surrounds the kidney.

Reprinted with permission, Cleveland Clinic Center for Medical Art & Photography © 2007–2014. All Rights Reserved.

**Table 8** Indications for Partial Nephrectomy (Nephron Sparing Surgery)

| Indication | Explanation | Examples |
|---|---|---|
| Absolute | To prevent complete loss of kidney function making patient dependent on dialysis | Tumor in both kidneys<br>Tumor in only functioning kidney, a "solitary kidney" |
| Relative | To preserve the function of a kidney threatened by other diseases | Diabetes<br>High blood pressure<br>Kidney stone disease<br>Recurrent urinary infections<br>Chronic kidney disease<br>Renal artery disease |
| Elective | To preserve long-term function of two otherwise normal kidneys not currently threatened by other systemic diseases | Tumors ≤ 4–7 cm and a normal kidney on the other side |

nephrectomies would absolutely result in dialysis; therefore, partial nephrectomy is a necessity. Relative indications occur in patients whose overall kidney function is currently or potentially compromised by other illnesses including diabetes, high blood pressure, kidney stones, chronic infections, lupus, or other disorders affecting kidney function. In these instances, removing the kidney may result in marginal remaining kidney function and a risk of imminent or subsequent dialysis.

"Elective" partial nephrectomy refers to removal of a kidney mass in a patient with two normal functioning kidneys. In such cases, kidney preservation is "elective" because removal of the entire kidney would not put the patient in immediate need of dialysis. Partial nephrectomy seeks to save as much kidney function as possible in case kidney problems such as diabetes or high blood pressure develop for any reason in the future.

Because it is more technically demanding, partial nephrectomy is underutilized in the management of RCC. Partial nephrectomy requires reconstruction of the kidney and is actually more challenging than radical nephrectomy. It can be associated with a slightly higher risk of bleeding, urinary leakage, infection, and poor healing of the reconstructed kidney. Hence, both the surgeon and patient assume additional risks to preserve the kidney. Fortunately most urine leaks close with conservative management such as a temporary kidney stent and time, and postoperative bleeding occurs in only about 1–2% of patients. The upside of partial nephrectomy can be substantial, saving kidney function and reducing the risk of needing dialysis in the future. It is important to ask your surgeon whether you are a candidate for partial nephrectomy and if not, why not.

There is a new system that surgeons have adopted now to estimate the complexity of a partial nephrectomy called the R.E.N.A.L. (radius, exophytic/endophytic properties, nearness of tumor to the collecting system or sinus in millimeters, anterior/posterior, location relative to polar lines) nephrometry score. In this system, several factors are scored to determine the difficulty and risk of a partial nephrectomy. The R.E.N.A.L. Nephrometry Score goes from a low of 4 to a high of 12. Patients with a score of 4, 5, or 6 are deemed "easy" with a low risk of complications. Nearly all of these tumors can be excised using a partial nephrectomy usually performed laparoscopically or robotically. Patients with a score of 7, 8, or 9 have an "intermediate" complexity and risk but most can still be treated with partial nephrectomy. Finally scores of 10, 11, or 12 are the most complex for partial nephrectomy with the highest risk of postoperative complications. Partial nephrectomies in these patients are usually performed via an open incision and should be reserved for those at risk of losing too much kidney function. These require an even higher level of surgical expertise and experience. Remember, in about 2–3% of patients, kidney cancer recurs in the opposite kidney and if the entire kidney was taken out several years before, this may seriously limit future options.

As with any clinical decision, the choice of a partial versus radical nephrectomy is always a risk versus benefit analysis. On the one hand, partial nephrectomies are more complicated and may be associated with a higher risk of postoperative problems, but on the other hand saving a portion of normal kidney may be in your overall best interest. Partial nephrectomies can be performed either openly or laparoscopically/robotically. Laparoscopic or robotic partial nephrectomy (**Figure 16**) is a technically demanding operation that was initially

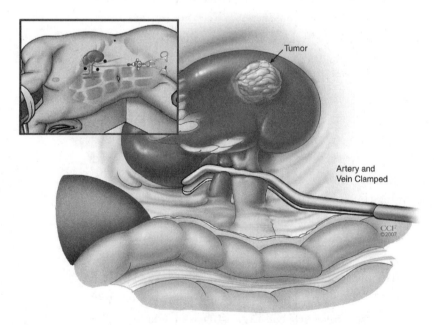

**Figure 16a** Schematic of laparoscopic/robotic partial nephrectomy. A vascular clamp occludes the renal vein and artery, blocking blood flow to and from the kidney.
Reprinted with permission, Cleveland Clinic Center for Medical Art & Photography © 2007–2014. All Rights Reserved.

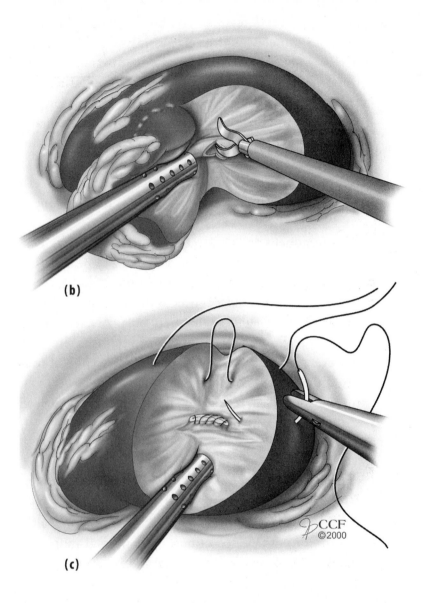

(b)

(c)

**Figure 16b,c** Scissors are then used to cut the tumor out of the kidney with a margin of normal tissue (b).

Entry into the collecting system is sewn closed to prevent a urine leak. Additional sutures are then placed to close the capsule, similar to the open surgical technique (c).

offered at only a few centers, but is being performed by more surgeons with each passing year. The choice depends not only on individual circumstances such as tumor size, location, prior surgeries, etc., but also on the surgeon's experience with complex kidney surgery. Moreover, you want to do your own risk-benefit analysis on the type of procedure being recommended. For example, if you have only one kidney, is the benefit of laparoscopy (smaller incisions, quicker recovery) worth the added risk of complications with your only kidney?

Your treatment decisions must be made with an understanding of the potential risks you will accept. Existing published data favors fewer complications and less risk with an open partial nephrectomy, and laparoscopic/robotic partial nephrectomy may be associated with a slightly greater amount of normal kidney tissue removed; however, this very much depends on the specifics of your case and your surgeon's skill set. In making this decision, many patients will read and get opinions by experienced and respected national surgical thought leaders.

## 48. What is an "elective" partial nephrectomy?

An "elective" partial nephrectomy refers to removal of the tumor with preservation of the normal kidney in the setting of two otherwise normal functioning kidneys, in situations in which a partial nephrectomy is not absolutely required. Although initially all kidney tumors were removed by radical nephrectomy, over time physicians realized that, for many patients, complete removal is unnecessary. This is similar to the evolution of other types of cancer surgeries such as radical mastectomy for breast cancer. We now know that many women with breast cancer can be effectively treated with a lumpectomy and radiation therapy, and the breast can be preserved. As thinking about kidney tumors became more refined, it was realized that the risk of a cancer recurrence for appropriately selected patients was not higher for partial nephrectomy.

Initial experience with partial nephrectomy began for absolute or relative indications. With greater collective experience, elective partial nephrectomy has become routine in an effort to preserve more functional kidney and reduce the risk of kidney failure on a long-term basis. Surgeons have been asking "Is there a tumor size cutoff at which the risk of recurrence or major complications is significantly higher for partial versus radical nephrectomy?"

The most widely accepted size cutoff for an elective partial nephrectomy is 4–7 cm. Large published surgical series demonstrate that if your tumor is < 4–7 cm, the likelihood of cure is the same regardless of whether the entire kidney, or just part of it, is removed. Size is not the only factor to be considered. Location is also important, as is a surgeon's experience. The more peripherally located a tumor, the easier it is to perform a partial nephrectomy and the fewer associated potential complications. The more central the tumor, the closer it is to vital structures of the kidney, the more difficult the partial nephrectomy. Here too, a surgeon's experience counts. What may be a difficult or impossible partial nephrectomy to one surgeon may be routine to another.

Several technical points should be emphasized regarding partial nephrectomies. First, the primary goal is the same as with radical nephrectomy, to remove the entire cancer. The surgeon may occasionally perform an intraoperative frozen section to be sure there is no residual tumor left behind. This means that the edge of the resection, or margin, is analyzed for the presence of cancer cells by a pathologist. If the margin is positive for cancer cells, he or she will generally remove more tissue. Secondly, the surgeon will need to reconstruct the remaining kidney. This requires expertise to reduce the risk of complications after the kidney has been reconstructed. The surgeon must also believe that the amount of remaining normal kidney tissue will contribute meaningfully to the patient's overall kidney function. Therefore, there is a strong element of experience in the preoperative and intraoperative decision-making process during complicated kidney cancer surgery.

Surgeons and patients must always consider the possibility of developing postoperative kidney insufficiency or failure after complete removal of a kidney. Although one kidney is usually sufficient for the remainder of a patient's life, you can never have too much normal kidney! Kidney stones, infection, high blood pressure, diabetes, and aging all can develop as the years go by and can have an adverse effect on overall kidney function. Saving maximal amounts of normal kidney is especially beneficial in younger patients with decades of life remaining.

Additionally, a patient who loses one kidney to cancer has a higher risk of developing cancer in the other kidney. Finally, since cancer patients are generally older, they may require more medications and are more likely to have or acquire diseases that affect kidney function. There are now compelling data that suggest a real functional benefit of preserving as much normal kidney as you can at the time of kidney cancer surgery. In this sense, elective partial nephrectomy is now becoming a standard of care rather than just an elective procedure.

## 49. What happens to the tumor after it is removed?

After the tumor is removed it is sent to the pathologist. Depending on the type of surgery, a quick pathologic analysis, or frozen section, may be performed. Here, the pathologist freezes a small section of tissue for immediate microscopic evaluation. Unlike with partial nephrectomy, frozen section is not usually performed following radical nephrectomy. After surgery, your physician may discuss the results of a frozen section; however, since frozen sections are "quick evaluations," they are not considered the final word. All removed tissues will undergo pathological processing including a detailed inspection, fixation, and staining for microscopic evaluation. This process may take several days. During this time, the pathologist will classify the type of tumor, the pathological extent (stage) of the tumor, and the grade of the tumor. Occasionally special pathological studies may be done including **immunohistochemistry** and **cytogenetic** analyses. These studies may aid the pathologist and the clinician in classifying the nature of the tumor and in recommending follow-up treatments or surveillance studies. Most pathological specimens are kept for several years in the department of pathology in case there is a need to go back and refer to the specimen again.

**Immuno-histochemistry**

Microscopic localization of specific antigens in tissues by staining with antibodies labeled with fluorescent pigmented material.

**Cytogenetic**

The branch of biology that deals with heredity and the cellular components such as chromosomes.

## 50. What is laparoscopy and how is it different from robotics?

Laparoscopy refers to the use of small instruments and telescopes (cameras that look inside the body) to access various compartments of the abdomen. Laparoscopic techniques have been available for kidney surgery for only the last 20–25 years. During laparoscopy, carbon dioxide gas is pumped into the abdomen through small channels called ports (think of them like thick straws which poke through the abdominal cavity). This creates a space between the abdominal wall and the intraabdominal organs. A camera is placed within one of the ports and working instruments in the others. There are three types of laparoscopic kidney surgery. The first is a **transabdominal** laparoscopy where you work through the front side of the abdomen. Here the working space is bigger; however, it requires mobilization of the intestines, which lie in front of the kidney. If a patient has had prior surgery and adhesions have formed, these will need to be addressed before the actual nephrectomy can begin.

**Transabdominal**

Across the abdominal wall or through the abdominal cavity.

The transperitoneal approach is the most commonly used. In the retroperitoneal approach, the port sites for the camera and working instruments are placed in the flank and back, enabling the surgeon to stay away from the bowels all together (**Figure 17**). This gives the most direct approach to the kidney and its blood vessels and is very useful in patients who have had extensive prior abdominal surgery. It is technically more challenging and many surgeons have not been trained in this approach. Finally, the hand-assist approach makes a slightly larger incision and allows the surgeon to insert his hand as an instrument. This is sometimes used for very large tumors or by less experienced laparoscopic surgeons.

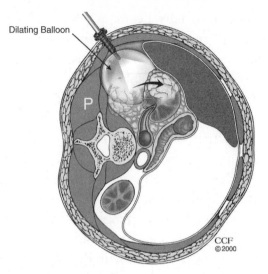

**Figure 17a** During retroperitoneal laparoscopic radical nephrectomy, balloon dilation of the space provides working room so that the vessels to the kidney are well visualized.

Reprinted with permission, Cleveland Clinic Center for Medical Art & Photography
© 2007–2014. All Rights Reserved.

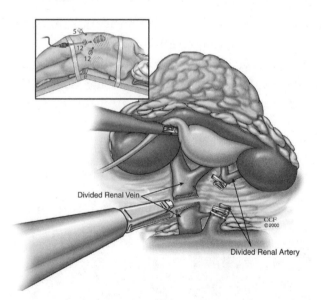

**Figure 17b** The vessels are then divided with clips and a stapling device, so that the kidney can be freed of all attachments and removed from the body.

Reprinted with permission, Cleveland Clinic Center for Medical Art & Photography
© 2007–2014. All Rights Reserved.

**Robotic**

See robot-assisted laparoscopic surgery.

**Robot-assisted laparoscopic surgery**

Some laparoscopic surgeries are performed with a robotic surgical system, and termed "robot-assisted laparoscopic" or "robotic" surgeries. The surgeon is involved from the start to finish, performing the surgery with the assistance of the surgical robot.

Many people have now heard of **"robotic"** surgery. **Robot-assisted laparoscopic surgery** is simply a fancy form of laparoscopy in which a robot is used to manipulate the working instruments. The surgeon sits at a console and dictates all of the movements; the robot just translates these movements into actions with the instruments in the body (**Figure 17c**). Robotics has two distinct advantages: first the picture is 3D and second the tools in the body are more flexible and therefore more easily manipulated. Some patients seem to believe that the robot automates or even performs the surgery. This is not true. The robot is only a tool but the surgeon and his/her experience remain the most important variable to how well the operation is performed. The surgeon doesn't program the robot to do the surgery, he/she actually manipulates the controls which the robot translates into the internal motion of the robotic arms.

A laparoscopic approach is considered the standard of care if radical nephrectomy is performed for most stage I and II kidney cancers. It should be used only by very experienced surgeons for stage III and IV disease. In expert hands and for carefully selected patients,

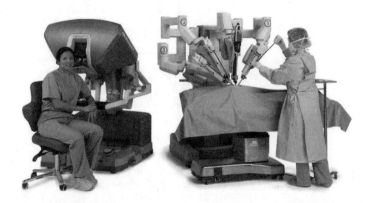

**Figure 17c** Surgeon Console/Patient Cart-da Vinci Si HD Surgical System.

©2014 Intuitive Surgical, Inc.

laparoscopy does not put a patient at higher risk for complications and has the added benefit of a shorter hospital stay and quicker recovery. In the absence of complicating factors such as tumor thrombus, massive tumors, or extensive lymph node enlargement, laparoscopy is safe and effective for radical nephrectomy.

If a partial nephrectomy is indicated, a laparoscopic or robotic approach is dependent on the size and location of the lesion as well as the surgeon's experience. Again, the **risk–benefit ratio** must be carefully evaluated when considering a laparoscopic or robotic partial nephrectomy.

While laparoscopy is an excellent approach for kidney tumor ablations—and it is extremely rare that open ablations need to be done—most ablations are now done percutaneously. If surgery is required or recommended a laparoscopic or robotic partial nephrectomy is considered the best approach for tumors otherwise amenable to ablation. Good clinical judgment suggests that if a surgeon is going to make an incision to approach the kidney tumor, the patient is better served by excising the tumor rather than ablating it.

**Risk–benefit ratio**

Counting the cost before making a decision, thinking of both the harms and benefits of acting and the chances that they will occur.

## 51. What is cryoablation?

The term "ablation" refers to destruction of a tumor without subsequent removal of the destroyed tissue. These procedures use various forms of energy to destroy the renal mass while attempting to preserve the adjacent normal kidney tissue. The advantage is that the surgery is less invasive and recovery times are shortened.

Cryoablation remains the most widely used and studied of ablative technologies for RCC. Renal cryoablation refers to the destruction of the kidney tumor by rapid freezing to a temperature below −40 degrees Celsius followed by rapid thawing of the tissue. This rapid freezing kills the cells directly by disrupting the cells' membranes and inner-cellular machinery while also starving the cells of blood flow, oxygen, and water. The rapid thawing further damages the lining of the tumor's blood vessels making subsequent tumor recovery highly improbable. The freeze thaw cycle is then repeated a second time to destroy any remaining cellular processes.

Renal cryoablation is most often performed percutaneously. A cryoprobe is inserted into the tumor under radiographic guidance. Argon gas is circulated through the probe and this part of the kidney is frozen, creating an "iceball," which then slowly expands. This iceball intentionally kills the tumor and a small surrounding rim of normal tissue (**Figure 18**). The size of the iceball can be monitored during this process to accurately control the extent of freezing and the amount of the kidney that is killed. Open cryoablation through an incision is uncommonly performed and is somewhat counterintuitive since it deprives the patient of its real benefit, which is to be minimally invasive.

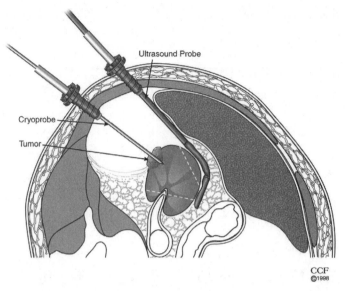

**Figure 18a** Cryosurgical ablation is performed by placement of a probe into the kidney tumor using ultrasound guidance. The tumor is then frozen to lethal temperatures along with a safe margin of normal kidney.

Reprinted with permission, Cleveland Clinic Center for Medical Art & Photography © 2007–2014. All Rights Reserved.

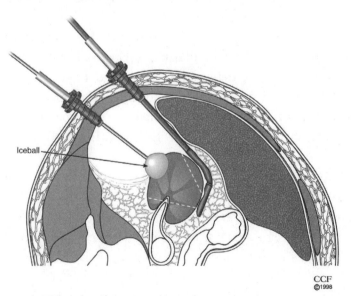

**Figure 18b** The size of the growing "iceball" is monitored continuously by ultrasound to make sure that the entire tumor is frozen.

Reprinted with permission, Cleveland Clinic Center for Medical Art & Photography © 2007–2014. All Rights Reserved.

As with any new approach, ask your urologist specifically about his/her personal experience as he/she usually works with the radiologist to perform ablative procedures. You should also ask the radiologist about his/her personal experience not only with the technique but also with managing its complications and with managing kidney cancer in general. It should be emphasized that doctors taking care of kidney cancer should not only be technicians, but should also have a vast knowledge and experience in taking care of all aspects of the disease, including its symptoms, behavior, and follow-up.

## 52. What is radiofrequency ablation (RFA)?

Radiofrequency ablation (RFA) is another energy-based technology used to destroy small kidney tumors without removing them. RFA uses alternating current to heat tissue thereby causing direct cell death and injury and eradication of the tumor's blood supply. The equipment for RFA consists of an alternating electric current generator, a probe to deliver the energy, and a radiographic or laparoscopic technique to guide probe placement. The majority of RFA procedures today are performed percutaneously under radiographic guidance (**Figure 19**).

In order to prevent overheating of the probe and damage to normal surrounding tissue, manufacturers of RFA probes use temperature sensors or impedance measurements to regulate flow of the electrical current. Other methods used to prevent overheating include internal cooling of the probe tip and use of pulsed electric current. None of these technologies has proven advantages over the others.

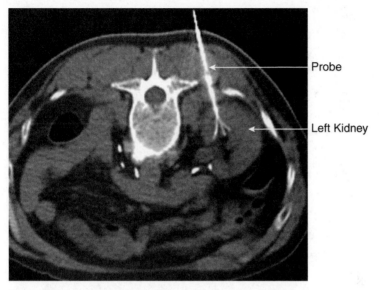

**Figure 19a** Radiofrequency ablation (RFA) can be performed percutaneously under radiographic guidance using MRI or CT.

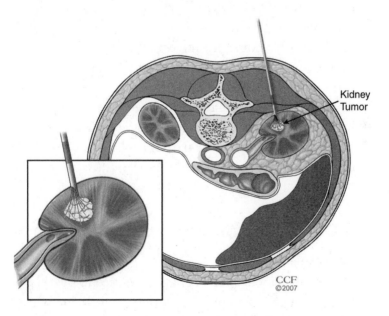

**Figure 19b** During RFA, a probe is placed directly into the tumor and then heated to lethal temperatures to destroy the tumor.

TREATMENT: LOCALIZED DISEASE

RFA has several limitations and potential disadvantages when compared to cryoablation. First, unlike cryoablation, where a distinct iceball is visible radiographically, RFA does not change the appearance of the lesion radiographically. This makes it more difficult to assess the extent of tissue destruction. Secondly, heat from an RFA probe dissipates into surrounding tissues. This "heat sink" effect may decrease the effectiveness of RFA and is problematic around blood vessels. Another potential disadvantage is that entire tumor kill is usually delayed and may not be complete for up to 30–120 days. Additionally, experimental animal models demonstrate that injury of the urinary collecting system is significantly higher with RFA than with cryoablation, so the risk of urine leakage from the treated kidney is theoretically higher. Finally, it may be more difficult to assess the long-term effects of RFA radiographically because microscopic tumor cells may be present despite a technically "successful" result. At this point in time cryoablation and RFA are best reserved for patients who are not good operative candidates due to advanced age or other medical problems. Patients who can tolerate surgery and are otherwise candidates for ablation should strongly consider surgical excision most often by partial nephrectomy, because excision has the best long-term proven track record.

## 53. What are the pros and cons of each of these ablation options?

Both cryoablation and RFA have been used to treat small kidney cancers. So how does a physician decide which is best for you? The practical answer is that many physicians have more experience with one option based upon their training; however, a critical review of the literature brings some important differences into perspective.

**Table 9** presents the pros and cons of surgical excision versus thermal ablation, and **Table 10** compares the two main forms of thermal ablation, cryosurgery or RFA.

It should be remembered that cryoablation of renal masses has been used for a longer time and therefore has been more intensely studied and scrutinized by urologic oncologists than RFA. This is not to suggest that RFA is inferior, but rather that the data for RFA of kidney cancers is less mature.

One final word about ablation is that it may require retreatment in 10–15% of cases. Moreover, while partial nephrectomy can be performed in patients who have failed ablation, it is technically very difficult. Therefore ablation should not be used in the young or in whom surgery would be the best initial treatment in experienced hands.

## 54. Can I just be observed? What are the risks of not actively seeking treatment for kidney cancer?

Delaying or refusing treatment is always an option for any patient as long as they are well informed about the risks of doing so. In years past, physicians rarely recommended observation for a variety of reasons: kidney cancer often cannot be salvaged if it progresses to metastatic disease; there was a misunderstanding about the risks associated with early-stage disease; and many physicians were concerned about medical/legal issues if the patient progressed and was no longer curable.

Currently, data continues to accumulate that quantify the risks of a "wait-and-see" approach in highly selected

**Table 9** Pros and Cons of Excision Versus Ablation

| | Excision (Radical or Partial Nephrectomy) | Ablation (Cryosurgery or RFA) |
|---|---|---|
| Appropriate tumor size | Any | <3 cm |
| Appropriate tumor location | Any | Peripheral |
| *Pathologic assessment* | | |
| • Of tissue | Complete | Biopsy |
| • Of margins | Complete | None |
| *Approach* | | |
| • Open technique | Yes | Almost never |
| • Laparoscopic | Yes | Yes (extremely rare) |
| • Percutaneous | No | Yes |
| Potential for blood loss | Moderate | Minimal |
| Risk of urine leak (fistula) | < 5% | < 2% |
| *Pain potential* | | |
| • Early | Moderate | Minimal |
| • Delayed | Minimal | Minimal |
| *Full recovery* | | |
| • Open technique | 4–6 weeks | Almost never done |
| • Laparoscopic | 2–3 weeks | 1–2 weeks (though this is almost never done) |
| • Percutaneous | Not done | 1 week |
| Reported long-term efficacy | 90–98% | 80–95% |

patients with small, early kidney cancer. Because early-stage kidney cancer is often diagnosed in asymptomatic elderly patients with other medical problems, clinicians will sometimes recommend observation to avoid treatment-associated risks.

In a recent review of all the published literature on the topic of untreated kidney masses, approximately one-third

**Table 10** Pros and Cons of Cryoablation Versus RFA

| | Cryoablation | Radio Frequency Ablation |
|---|---|---|
| Method of ablation | Freezing to −40°C or below | Heating tissue to lethal temperatures |
| Most frequent technique | Laparoscopic = Percutaneous | Percutaneous > Laparoscopic |
| First reported use in kidney cancer | 1995 | 1998 |
| Real time monitoring of ablative area? | Yes | No |
| Visual changes during treatment | Yes | No |
| Time to kill cancer cells | < 48 hours | 3–120 days |
| Risk of recurrent or residual disease | 3.0% | 13.4% |
| Adjacent organ injury | Possible | Possible |
| Treatment time | Short | Short |
| Risk of bleeding | Low | Low |
| Percent size decrease of ablated lesion | More with time (75% at 3 years) | Minimal |
| Percent of tumors not visible radiographically 3 years after ablation | 32% | Rare |
| Is re-ablation possible? | Yes | Yes |
| Is partial nephrectomy possible if ablation fails? | Yes | Yes |
| Is partial nephrectomy difficult if necessary? | Yes | Yes |
| Reported mean % of disease-free survival | 85–95% | 80–90% |

of small (< 3 cm) kidney tumors did not increase in size over a median of nearly 3 years, and those that grew tended to have a very slow growth rate between 2–5 mm per year. Moreover, the risk of spread or metastasis in patients being observed was relatively low (< 5%) (**Table 11**). However, there are some important caveats to keep in mind when considering these results. First, patients in these series were very carefully selected

**Table 11**  Key Facts Regarding Active Surveillance of Small Renal Masses

- The majority of enhancing renal masses are renal cell carcinoma (kidney cancer) until proven otherwise
- There is a loose correlation between renal tumor size and the likelihood that it represents cancer
  - As many as 25–30% of renal masses < 2–3 cm may be benign
  - More than 85% of renal masses > 3 cm are malignant
- There are no reliable predictors of which renal tumors will grow under active surveillance
- The average growth rate of an incidental small renal tumor is 2–3 mm per year during the first 3 years of follow-up
- The risk of a small incidental renal mass progressing to metastatic disease under active surveillance appears to be small, particularly in the absence of radiographic growth
- Active surveillance is best indicated in the elderly and/or infirm patient with asymptomatic small renal masses
- Approximately 30% of incidental small renal masses show zero grow when followed radiographically for 3 years
- Limitations regarding active surveillance data exist, although in well selected patients observation is a reasonable choice
- Patients and physicians who choose active surveillance assume a calculated risk
- Active surveillance or watching a kidney tumor is rarely a good long-term option in patients with a life expectancy > 10 years

(anyone with a potentially aggressive appearing tumor had surgery); most series were retrospective and thus less reliable; not all patients had biopsy-proven kidney cancer; most patients were elderly or had other medical risks; and the average follow-up of these lesions was only about 3 years. These considerations must be kept in mind when weighing out a course of active surveillance. Moreover, when an informed patient elects observation, both the patient and his/her family must be willing to accept the risk that his or her individual tumor may act more aggressively, that it may progress to an incurable stage, and the patient must be willing to live with this risk.

Nonetheless, in elderly patients, particularly those with considerable surgical risks, a judicious period of surveillance for tumors < 3 cm with treatment for those patients whose tumor demonstrates growth is a potential option. It is important that patients electing observation be followed diligently by a urologic oncologist with a broad experience observing these tumors and knowing when to intervene.

## 55. How will I be followed after a radical nephrectomy?

After surgery you will receive your final pathology report. Based on this report you will be assigned a stage. Your follow-up will then be based on a stage-specific risk of recurrence following radical nephrectomy. Follow-up will include periodic history, physical examination, and routine lab tests. These may include compete blood counts and serum chemistries to evaluate the ability of your remaining kidney to filter wastes and a urinalysis to determine if your remaining kidney is wasting protein. Finally, your doctor will order radiographic tests to determine whether your cancer has silently returned.

Between 50% and 80% of kidney cancer recurrences are asymptomatic, so the most important tests are radiographic surveys, typically including a chest X-ray, CT scan, MRI, or ultrasound. Because the likelihood of recurrence depends largely on your initial tumor stage, the follow-up is often tailored to your stage. This is termed stage-specific surveillance. Low-risk patients do not need CT scans very often and their follow-up is greatly simplified. Microscopic metastases that are not visible and cannot be identified at the time of surgery are typically responsible for most cancer recurrences.

For many patients this can be a real shock and surprise and they will often wonder how this can happen because the main cancer has been removed and everything pointed toward a cure. But in some patients small nests of cancer cells have escaped the kidney prior to surgery and set up camp at other sites in the body, such as the lungs or bones. Preoperative X-rays and CT scans cannot pick up such microscopic disease, the final pathology may suggest confined disease, and all signs may point in a positive direction. However, as the months and years pass, these microscopic nests can grow and pick up momentum, and eventually start to cause trouble.

If cancer does return, it typically returns as kidney cancer cells located in other organs such as the lungs, liver, lymph nodes, or adrenals. Less commonly, it can recur in the bones or brain. Therefore chest and abdomen imaging are most important, but again this is tailored to each individual patient's stage and risk. The National Comprehensive Cancer Network (NCCN) and American Urologic Association (AUA) have established guidelines for follow-up that should be familiar to your physician.

Although recurrences from RCC can occur decades after surgery, this is uncommon. Most recurrences are found within the first 1–3 years. Your doctor will most likely recommend more frequent studies in the initial years following surgery and fewer in the ensuing years. After an initial 5-year period, the risk of recurrences diminishes. Unfortunately, this risk is never completely zero, but in most patients the 5-year cancer-free mark is a major and important milestone.

## 56. How will I be followed after a partial nephrectomy?

The same principles of stage-specific surveillance following radical nephrectomy hold true following partial nephrectomy. A recurrence in the "remnant kidney" is deemed a local recurrence and the risk of this developing depends on the initial stage. After partial nephrectomy for localized disease, the risk of a local recurrence is sufficiently low that follow-up is the same as with radical nephrectomy. For patients with microscopic or major venous involvement (stage III), the likelihood of recurrence in the remnant kidney is higher. In these cases CTs or MRIs are performed more frequently (usually every 6 months) for the first year or two, then at least yearly after this.

A local recurrence in the remnant kidney is often treated with surgery to remove the remnant kidney so early diagnosis is imperative. Surveillance CT or MRI following partial nephrectomy should ideally be performed before and after intravenous contrast. A mass within the kidney is suspicious for a new or recurrent cancer if it enhances (lights up with contrast). This suggests increased blood flow in and out of the tumor, and indicates malignancy.

After partial nephrectomy, patients with compromised kidney function may need follow-up with the surgeon and a **nephrologist** (medical kidney specialist). A nephrologist can help devise an appropriate medical strategy to optimize the function of the remaining kidney and prevent or delay progressive kidney failure. This may reduce or delay the need for dialysis in some patients.

**Nephrologist**

A physician subspe-
cialized in manag-
ing non-surgical
kidney disease, who
is board-certified in
internal medicine
and nephrology.

## 57. How will I be followed after cryoablation or RFA?

Since ablation is reserved for small, low-risk, stage I tumors, follow-up after ablation is tailored toward determining whether there is residual or recurrent disease within the ablation bed. The development of metastases in properly selected patients after ablation is uncommon. Success after ablation means the mass should not enhance with intravenous contrast. If it convincingly enhances, this suggests residual or recurrent tumor that may require a reablation or excision.

It is not always easy to determine whether there is enhancement postablation because inflammation or blood may obscure the view. A well-performed CT or MRI of the kidney is the best way to determine enhancement. These studies will also evaluate the presence of disease in other locations within the abdomen. The importance of a well-performed and properly interpreted scan cannot be overemphasized. Some general radiologists may lack the experience to perform or read scans following ablation. You must be your own advocate and insist on properly performed studies or be sure you are seeing a kidney cancer specialist.

While lack of enhancement is generally considered the final goal after ablation, it has been demonstrated that despite failure to enhance, biopsy of some lesions, particularly following RFA, may show residual microscopic tumor cells. Until long-term data are available following ablative technologies, these techniques should be considered less definitive than excision. Until a large number of patients have been treated with these modalities and followed for many years, we will not know whether these less-invasive treatments are really as effective as we hope they will be.

# PART SIX

# *Treatment: Locally Advanced Disease*

What is the treatment for locally advanced (stage III) kidney cancer?

How is a tumor thrombus removed?

What if the tumor thrombus goes into the heart?

*More*\*...

\*Words that may not be familiar to you are included in the glossary.
We have highlighted them in **bold** when they are first used in this book.

## 58. What is the treatment for locally advanced (stage III) kidney cancer?

As many as 4 in 10 patients will present with stage III or IV kidney cancer, and these stages of disease are a major challenge. In these patients the tumor extends outside of the kidney, into the adrenal gland, lymph nodes, or invades into the renal vein or inferior vena cava (tumor thrombus). For such patients, the primary goal is to remove all identifiable disease in a safe and effective manner. For patients with lymph node involvement, this means removing all possible involved lymph nodes, including adjacent lymph nodes that appear normal. For patients with venous involvement, this means removing the entire tumor thrombus. For patients with disease into the adrenal or fat around the kidney, this requires removing all the surrounding fat and the adrenal gland.

Many patients with locally advanced disease worry about their risk of recurrence. This is a real concern because between 20% of "intermediate-risk" and 70% of patients with "high-risk" kidney cancer may recur within 5 years. There are many factors to take into consideration when trying to predict recurrence in patients who have undergone surgery (**Table 12**). In an effort to better evaluate a patient's risk of recurrence, tables, algorithms, and predictive statistical models or **nomograms** that combine several of these risk factors are available to help predict the likelihood of recurrence (**Figure 20**). It should be mentioned that interpretation of these data requires insight into the disease and the methods used to derive the data. The numbers predicted by the nomograms should be used as a guide rather than an absolute number, because the complexity of each patient's situation cannot be wholly reflected in tables or prediction tools. Following surgery for locally advanced disease, additional systemic therapies may be recommended.

*Many patients with locally advanced disease worry about their risk of recurrence.*

**Nomogram**

A predictive model that estimates the likelihood of a given outcome (such as recurrence of cancer or death due to cancer) based on specific characteristics of an individual patient and his or her cancer. Nomograms are intended to be user-friendly versions of complicated predictive models, and they are often available for doctors and patients in paper-based formats or even online. www.cancernomograms.com is a website that allows simple input of clinical characteristics into kidney cancer nomograms that then allows the user to estimate risk of a given outcome (see Figure 20).

**Table 12** Prognostic Factors for RCC

| Anatomical | Histological | Clinical | Molecular |
|---|---|---|---|
| Tumor size | Nuclear grade | Localized symptoms | CA IX |
| Tumor extension | Histological subtype | Performance status | VEGF, VGFR |
| Adrenal gland involvement | Presence of sarcomatoid features | Cachexia | Insulin-like growth factor-1 |
| Vascular involvement | Presence of histological necrosis | Thrombocytosis | HIF |
| Lymph node involvement | Collecting system invasion | Anemia | Ki-67 |
| Distant metastasis | | Hypercalcemia | PCNA |
| | | Elevated alkaline phosphatase | p53 |
| | | Elevated C-reactive protein | PTEN |
| | | Elevated erythrocyte sedimentation rate | BAP1 |
| | | | Aberrant DNA methylation |

## 59. *How is a tumor thrombus removed?*

Removal of the tumor thrombus is surgical and based primarily on the highest level to which it extends. With relatively rare exceptions, removal of a kidney tumor associated with a thrombus requires a radical nephrectomy. It is uncommon for a partial nephrectomy to be done in the setting of a vena caval thrombus but occasionally it is possible when the situation arises in a solitary kidney. Additionally, the majority of renal cell carcinoma (RCC) cases associated with thrombus are

**Figure 20**  QR code of Fox Chase nomogram web site. Visit http://labs.fccc.edu/nomograms/ for more information.

removed via an open technique. Laparoscopy or robotics can be used only for limited thrombus involving primarily the kidney vein and not the vena cava. The physicians must determine the level of the thrombus prior to surgery to plan everything to be as safe as possible. There are a number of tests for this:

- **Venogram**: In this test, dye is injected into a vein and pictures are taken to identify the tumor thrombus. It is generally the most invasive test and also gives the least amount of anatomic detail. It has largely been replaced by other, less invasive tests and is now used only in very special circumstances.
- **CT scan**: While a CT scan may suggest the presence of a thrombus, it traditionally did not provide the anatomic detail necessary to determine the uppermost extent of the thrombus. However, the newest, most modern CT scanners can do this and are now considered a great test for this purpose.
- **MRI scan**: The MRI scan is one of the most sensitive tests for detection of a tumor thrombus and

**Venogram**

An X-ray of the veins produced by venography.

to define its uppermost extent. Typically this test is ordered as a *magnetic resonance venogram* (MRV). This is a technically difficult test to perform and many radiology centers are not well suited to perform it well. It is difficult to obtain a good MRV in an open MRI so this "shortcut" tends to be counterproductive. It is imperative that the MRV be performed properly to maximize the information obtained.

- **Intraoperative ultrasound (IOUS)**: In the operating room, many surgeons will use IOUS to identify or better confirm the extent of the thrombus. This can be performed either by placing the ultrasound probe directly on the vena cava or, even more sensitively, by performing a **transesophageal echocardiogram (TEE)**, which can visualize the vena cava all the way into the heart.

The surgical approach is dictated by the extent of the tumor thrombus; therefore, your surgeon would be very wise to accurately image the thrombus just prior to embarking on this highly complex surgery (typically a repeat imaging study is performed a day or two prior to surgery). Extraction of a tumor thrombus can be a life-threatening operation and should be done only by highly trained experts in kidney cancer surgery. Options for removal of most tumor thrombi (below the liver and heart) include complete control and occlusion or blockage of the vena cava followed by tumor extraction (**Figure 21**). If a highly trained urological oncologist is not available, a vascular surgeon should be involved. Occasionally the tumor thrombus invades the wall of the vena cava. In these cases, a portion of the vena cava may need to be **resected** (surgically cut out) and/or reconstructed.

**Intraoperative ultrasound (IOUS)**

Intraoperative ultrasound (IOUS) is a dynamic imaging modality that provides interactive and timely information during surgical procedures.

**Transesophageal echocardiogram (TEE)**

A technique used to visualize the heart and major blood vessels. In this version of echocardiography, the probe is placed inside the esophagus and for that reason is done when the person is asleep (under anesthesia).

**Resect**

To remove or excise tissue or part (or all) of an organ.

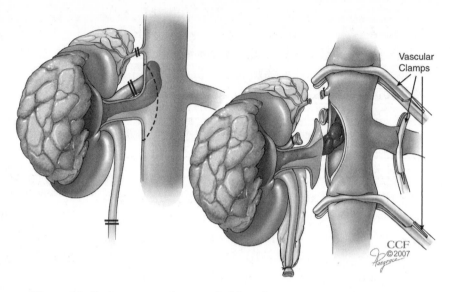

**Figure 21** Nephrectomy with removal of thrombus in vena cava. The ureter, renal artery, and vessels to the adrenal gland are identified and divided. The kidney is then attached to the body only by the renal vein containing the tumor thrombus. Vascular control of the opposite renal vein and the vena cava above and below this level is obtained prior to opening the vena cava and removing the thrombus. Suture repair of the defect in the vena cava is then performed and the vascular clamps are removed to complete the procedure.

Fortunately, while this surgery is technically complex, most patients with tumor thrombus can do very well after surgery and the presence of a tumor thrombus is often not associated with metastases. Overall, about 50% of these patients can be cured with a careful and comprehensive surgical approach.

## 60. What if the tumor thrombus goes into the heart?

Occasionally a tumor thrombus will extend above the liver veins (level 3) and/or into the heart (level 4). When this occurs, the stakes for removal are even higher. In these cases, bypass surgery may be required for safe removal of the tumor thrombus. The urologic oncologist, with a vascular or cardiac surgeon, will prepare for removal of the kidney and isolate all the necessary vasculature. The vascular or cardiac surgeon will then open the chest and put the patient on cardiac bypass. There are two different types of bypass; the first is termed veno-veno bypass in which the blood is shunted through a conduit around the tumor thrombus so that it can be removed without massive hemorrhage. The second type of bypass involves a classic cardiac bypass where the blood is removed and routed to a bypass machine. In these cases the patient's body will be cooled down to decrease metabolism rates and oxygen requirements. This is termed hypothermic circulatory arrest where the blood is temporarily removed from the body to provide a bloodless field. This is very similar to the bypass protocol that is used for heart surgery. The tumor thrombus is then quickly removed, the vena cava is sutured closed, and circulation is reestablished. The higher the tumor thrombus, the more technically demanding the surgery, and the greater the associated risks. Despite these risks, in most cases the tumor thrombus can be safely removed, even if it extends into the right atrium of the heart. Many of these patients can enjoy an excellent longer-term outcome.

## 61. What is the treatment of enlarged lymph nodes?

Mild enlargement of nearby lymph nodes (< 2.0 cm) may be associated with inflammation or cancer, and neither CT nor MRI is able to make this distinction in a reliable manner. In these cases, the lymph nodes are usually removed with the tumor. Larger lymph nodes are usually malignant, and again should be removed at the time of the nephrectomy if possible.

The pattern of lymph node spread in kidney cancer is unpredictable. Lymph node involvement in kidney cancer can be in the region of the affected kidney, along the aorta or vena cava, or in the chest or pelvis. In most patients it is not routine to remove all of these lymph nodes, although recent data suggest there may be a true advantage to extended lymph node removal in selected patients.

## 62. Why are adjacent organs sometimes removed?

In the case of locally advanced kidney cancer, nearby organs are sometimes involved by the tumor or tumor-associated inflammation and must be removed in part or in total. This is sometimes true for the adrenal gland or portions of the colon, liver, spleen, or pancreas that have been invaded by the tumor. In these cases, the surgeon may attempt to remove all visible tumor safely and effectively, which may require the expertise of a colorectal or liver/pancreatic surgeon. Fortunately, segments of colon, liver, and/or pancreas can often be removed with relatively few side effects. Kidney cancer is still best cured surgically, by removing all the cancer, and this sometimes requires a more extensive dissection with removal of adjacent organs.

Rarely, the need to remove a "bystander" organ occurs. This is especially true for portions of the diaphragm and/or spleen. Although these are not organs that typically become involved with kidney cancer, they may be inflamed and attached to the tumor and therefore require removal. In the case of partial removal of the diaphragm, it is usually possible to reconstruct this muscle and this rarely impacts the patient's breathing. If the spleen is removed, you may need to receive a yearly vaccination to prevent certain types of pneumonias that are more common in patients without a spleen.

## 63. What is an adjuvant treatment?

After surgery, your doctor will counsel you about the risks of recurrence. As discussed above these risks can be fairly well estimated using statistical models. Even in the best of circumstances there is always some risk of recurrence given the unpredictable nature of cancer.

Your physician may decide to use a predictive algorithm to determine the risk of recurrence in your specific circumstances. Based on this information, patients often want to know if there is anything they can do to decrease the risk of a recurrence. If your tumor is deemed intermediate or high risk and your chances of recurrence are relatively high, you may be offered adjuvant therapy. Adjuvant therapy refers to systemic therapies given relatively soon after surgery in the absence of clinical or radiographic disease in an effort to reduce the risk of recurrence. The concept is that if there is a small number of circulating microscopic metastatic cells, perhaps they can be killed while their numbers are low. These treatments are given "prophylactically" to *prevent* recurrence down the road. A classic example is a woman with breast cancer involving the lymph nodes, which is typically treated with chemotherapy after surgery even though the surgery appears to have rendered her disease-free. But we know that she is at risk because the cancer is showing aggressive tendencies, and the chemotherapy

*Your physician may decide to use a predictive algorithm to determine the risk of recurrence in your specific circumstances.*

is given as an "adjuvant" treatment to try to optimize the patient's chances long term.

Many, many adjuvant studies have been done after surgery for RCC. These have included the use of hormones, radiation, vaccines, immune-boosting cytokines, chemotherapy, and combination therapies. Unfortunately, to date no adjuvant strategies have proven effective for kidney cancer—none have improved the outcomes compared to close follow-up alone. Therefore, most patients with intermediate or high-risk kidney cancer take a wait-and-see approach or enroll in a clinical adjuvant kidney cancer trial.

Multiple new therapies for advanced kidney cancer have been introduced (see **Parts Seven**, **Eight**, and **Nine**) and many of these treatments have been or are being tested in the adjuvant setting using clinical trials. It is important for patients to understand that prospective clinical trials are conducted because it is unknown whether these medications will actually work in the adjuvant setting, or whether their risks or side effects will outweigh their benefits. These national trials are carefully reviewed and monitored by expert clinicians, academics, researchers, governmental agencies, and patient advocates to optimize patient safety and ensure fairness. All of these trials have a control or **placebo** arm for comparative purposes. Without this design we would never be able to determine whether the new treatment is actually working, and patients must know that they may be randomized to the placebo.

**Placebo**

A sugar pill that is given in clinical trials in order to help determine whether the effect seen with the real medication is due to the treatment itself or due to other reasons (placebo effect).

In addition, since there can be bias introduced if an investigator knows which medication (or placebo) you are taking, most physicians and patients are blinded to which treatment you are receiving. There are many other built-in contingencies for clinical trials including periodic safety monitoring, early termination clauses if the medicine is found to be highly effective, and ways that your doctor can find out which medication you are taking if problems arise. Moreover, some patients consider clinical trials with a placebo to be risky because they won't know if they receive the control (placebo) treatment. However, it should be clearly understood that if a patient with high-risk kidney cancer chooses not to participate in a clinical trial, they are essentially putting themselves on the "placebo" by choosing no treatment.

Clinical trials can be conducted and sponsored by individual hospitals, groups of hospitals, the pharmaceutical industry, and/or the National Cancer Institute (NCI) via the cooperative cancer group setting. The NCI has divided the country into several large collaborative groups. Clinical trials constantly open and close, and a listing of pertinent current clinical trials can be found at *www.clinicaltrials.gov*. For more information about clinical trials, please see **Part Ten**.

# PART SEVEN

# Treatment: Metastatic Disease

What are the treatment options for metastatic kidney cancer (stage IV)?

What is the prognosis for patients with metastatic kidney cancer?

Should I have a debulking nephrectomy?

*More*\*...

*Words that may not be familiar to you are included in the glossary. We have highlighted them in **bold** when they are first used in this book.

## 64. What are the treatment options for metastatic kidney cancer (stage IV)?

There are many different treatment options for kidney cancer that is metastatic, which means the kidney cancer cells have spread outside of the kidney to distant organs such as lung, bone, or brain (**Table 13**). These collections of kidney cancer cells are called metastases and are often detected by imaging studies, such as X-rays, CT scans, or bone scans. These studies cannot detect individual kidney cancer cells or small nests of cells. However, they can detect metastatic tumors that are larger than 1 cm in diameter, which corresponds to about one-half of an inch.

Even after the kidney cancer cells travel to other organs, they are still kidney cancer cells and are treated as such. Surgery to remove the primary kidney tumor should be considered if this has not already been done (see Question 66). Afterward, systemic therapy (meaning therapy that goes all over the body) should be received. This could consist of immunotherapy (designed to stimulate the body's immune system to fight the cancer), targeted therapy (therapy directed against specific protein targets that are related to the cancer), and/or participation in a clinical trial. Details of these options will be discussed in following questions.

There are also treatments that can be directed at kidney cancer that has spread to specific locations. For example, it is occasionally of benefit for a patient with a single, small metastasis in the lung or a local recurrence of cancer within the kidney to have surgical resection of the metastasis (metastasectomy). For bone metastases that cause significant pain, radiation therapy can play a role. For brain lesions, stereotactic radiation (focused radiation to just the tumor) can relieve neurologic symptoms and control tumor growth at that location. But these are special circumstances that will not apply to most patients with metastatic kidney cancer.

## 65. What is the prognosis for patients with metastatic kidney cancer?

One of the first questions that come to mind for patients with advanced cancer is, "How long do I have to live?" Historically, the average survival time for metastatic kidney cancer patients was about 12–14 months. The newer targeted drugs that are described below can lengthen this time, with recent trials showing an average survival for all patients of almost 2.5 years. For each cancer patient, the time course can be extremely variable, ranging from just a few months to several years. Several factors have been identified that can influence the outcome for individual patients (**Table 14**). For instance, patients who are still very active and functional tend to live longer on average. Their cancer has not impacted their lives as much, suggesting that the cancer may not be as aggressive, and they are better able to tolerate therapy. These patients with good "performance status" will tend to live longer than those whose disease is already knocking them out. However, even the factors listed in Table 14 cannot accurately predict the exact outcome for an individual patient, but rather they give a doctor and patient a general idea of the outcome for a group of patients with similar disease features.

Patients who respond to therapy will tend to live longer, and this is no surprise. However, factors that predict which patients will respond to therapy and what is the best treatment for any given patient are not yet available. A small subset of metastatic kidney cancer patients

**Table 13** Treatments for Metastatic Kidney Cancer

| Type of Treatment | Specific Treatment | Summary |
|---|---|---|
| Surgery | Nephrectomy (cytoreductive) | Kidney tumor is removed in order to facilitate other systemic treatments by reducing tumor burden (debulking) |
| | Metastasectomy | Removal of single or limited number of metastases with the intention of cure or relief of symptoms; common sites include adrenal gland, lung, abdominal, bone and brain metastases |
| Immunotherapy | Interleukin-2 (IL-2) | High-dose IL-2 is a potentially toxic regimen tolerated only by the most physically fit patients |
| | | Provides an opportunity for complete cure, but complete remissions are only seen in about 5% of patients. Overall response rate 14–25% |
| | Inhibition of check point control | Replaces the natural barriers that hold back the immune system so that it can be activated to fight the tumor more effectively |

*Targeted Molecular Therapy*

| | | |
|---|---|---|
| Anti-angiogenic agents | Sutent® (sunitinib) | Prevents the effects of the binding of VEGF to its receptor, so that VEGF is no longer active |
| | | 70–75% of patients will have tumors get smaller as a result of taking the drug |
| | Votrient ® (pazopanib) | Prevents the effects of the binding of VEGF to its receptor, so that VEGF is no longer active |
| | | 70–75% of patients will have tumors get smaller as a result of taking the drug |

| Type of Treatment | Specific Treatment | Summary |
|---|---|---|
| Anti-angiogenic agents (*continued*) | Nexavar® (sorafenib) | Prevents the effects of the binding of VEGF to its receptor, so that VEGF is no longer active |
| | | Tumor shrinkage in 70–75% of patients; overall response rate of 2–10% |
| | Inlyta® (axitinib) | Prevents the effects of the binding of VEGF to its receptor, so that VEGF is no longer active |
| | | Tumor shrinkage in 70–75% of patients; overall response rate of 19% |
| | Avastin® (bevacizumab) | Binds VEGF and inactivates it, preventing VEGF from stimulating new blood vessel growth |
| | | Tumor shrinkage in 70% of patients; overall response rate of 10-13% as monotherapy and 26-31% in combination with interferon |
| mTOR inhibitors | Torisel® (temsirolimus) | Blocks pathways inside the cell that prevent new blood vessel growth and tumor cell multiplication |
| | | Tumor shrinkage in 35% of patients; overall response rate of 19% |
| | Afinitor® (everolimus) | Blocks pathways inside the cell that prevent new blood vessel growth and tumor cell multiplication |
| | | Tumor shrinkage in 35% of patients; overall response rate of 1–5% |
| Chemotherapy | Multiple agents | Success rates have been very low with previous agents, but new agents are still being tested to try to find an active regimen; overall response rates of 4–5% |
| Radiation Therapy | | Used to treat brain metastases or painful metastases to the bones |

Overall response rates refer to the proportion of patients experiencing a complete response (100% reduction in tumor burden) or partial response (>30% reduction in tumor burden).

**Table 14** Prognostic Factors for Advanced Kidney Cancer

| |
|---|
| Performance Status: general level of well being/ability to perform daily tasks; a better performance status means the patient is more likely to respond to treatment |
| Time from first diagnosis of kidney cancer to development of metastases; a longer time is better because this means that the cancer is more indolent or slow growing |
| Hemoglobin level; normal is better |
| Lactate dehydrogenase level (blood protein); lower is better |
| Blood calcium level; normal is better |

(5–10%) can experience long-term survival (more than 5 years) either because of indolent (slow-growing) disease and/or a complete response to therapy. It is important that you ask your doctor to give you information about your specific prognosis so that you can know as much as possible about what might happen in the future.

## 66. Should I have a debulking nephrectomy?

Debulking or cytoreductive nephrectomy refers to surgery to remove the primary kidney tumor even though the tumor cells have already spread to other parts of the body (e.g., the lungs). This is not a curative procedure; the metastatic cancer sites are left behind, and the patient will still require additional systemic therapies. However, two studies have shown that cytoreductive nephrectomy can prolong survival by an average of 4–6 months. The rationale behind this procedure is that it can have a number of potential benefits:

- It reduces the total burden of disease and may thereby improve the likelihood that the remaining

metastatic tumors will respond to systemic treatments—the full treatment effect is then concen-
trated on the metastases.

- It eliminates the primary source of metastases—
remember that all of the metastases originally
came from the tumor in the kidney.

- There is also a theory that the primary tumor in the
kidney may secrete proteins into the bloodstream
that promote growth of the metastases or that tone
down the immune system—removal of the primary
tumor then will reverse these ill effects.

However, the potential benefits of a cytoreductive
nephrectomy must be weighed against the risk of surgery for each individual patient and the time required
for hospitalization and rehabilitation. In addition, some
patients (about 5–10%) will not recover adequately from
the surgery to allow them to receive systemic therapy,
and these patients tend to do poorly.

So, while a cytoreductive nephrectomy may benefit
many patients, it should not be done indiscriminately.
The best candidates for this procedure are patients
who are otherwise healthy and active (good performance status), have kidney tumors that can be removed
safely, and have most of their overall tumor burden in
the kidney. Future studies may aid in determining the
optimal use and timing of surgery.

## 67. Can other sites of disease be removed surgically?

If kidney cancer is still primarily a surgical disease, why
not just remove all of the metastases? The reason is that
there are limits to what surgery can do and most patients

with advanced kidney cancer have too many sites of disease or the disease is in very sensitive locations that are not amenable to surgical resection. In these patients, surgery would not be compatible with survival or they would be left with such poor quality of life that life would not be worth living.

However, a minority of patients with metastatic kidney cancer has only one or a few metastases and surgery can be considered in an effort to render them disease-free. Removal of these metastases is known as metastasectomy. This is an aggressive approach that should be considered only under special circumstances. Remember, it generally does not make sense to remove only part of the cancer, as cancer left behind still requires treatment. Also, CT scans only visualize large collections of tumor cells. There are often other cancer cells elsewhere that can't be seen on a scan. The site(s) of metastatic disease must be limited in number (usually just one or perhaps a few), limited in size, and the metastases must be in a surgically-accessible location. Some tumors cannot be resected or surgically removed safely. For instance, if the tumor is in certain areas of the brain or encasing a vital blood vessel it often cannot be removed safely—the patient would not survive or the risks of severe complications would be too high.

In general, the patients who are the best candidates for metastasectomy for kidney cancer have had a long period of time between removal of the primary tumor and the development of metastatic sites (generally greater than 1–2 years). In these patients the disease is more indolent (slow growing) and this likely contributes to the good outcomes in this subgroup of patients. Patients with lung metastases tend to do better than those with liver or bone metastases, and all of these factors must be taken into account. Yet even in the best of circumstances, only one out of every three patients who undergoes metastasectomy will remain cancer free. Most patients are found to have additional metastases as the months and years go by, and they are not cured of cancer. In these patients the metastasis was only the "tip of the iceberg," and their hidden micrometastatic disease ends up declaring itself.

## 68. Is chemotherapy an option?

Chemotherapy is used for most advanced cancers, why not kidney cancer? The reality is that kidney cancer does not appear to be very sensitive to chemotherapy. In fact, kidney cancer is considered the prototype of the chemorefractory cancer. Almost all chemotherapy drugs have been tested against this cancer and none have been particularly effective. In addition, several combinations of chemotherapeutic drugs have been tested, also with discouraging results.

There are a few chemotherapeutic agents that have limited activity (10–15% response rates) in kidney cancer. These include fluorouracil (5-FU), Gemzar (gemcitabine), and Adriamycin (doxorubicin). Combination of these agents with each other and with newer agents is underway, and research in this field continues with the hope that a more active agent or protocol will be found in the future.

Overall, when one considers the potential side effects of chemotherapy and the relatively low response rates, it is understandable that chemotherapy is not one of the main treatments for advanced kidney cancer at this point in time.

## 69. Is hormonal therapy an option?

Hormonal therapy is one of the mainstays for the treatment of patients with advanced prostate cancer. Can it play a role for patients with metastatic kidney cancer? Unfortunately, the answer is *no*. Hormonal therapy refers to treatments that alter the hormonal environment within the body to combat cancer, and one such treatment is Megace (medroxyprogesterone).

Megace was used historically to treat metastatic kidney cancer patients and it was originally thought to be helpful. However, when it was studied carefully it was found to be of very limited effectiveness for the majority of patients. Megace can stimulate the appetite and is still used in some patients with kidney cancer who are suffering from anorexia, although even in this setting its efficacy is debatable. Although other forms of cancer do respond to hormone treatment, kidney cancer does not, and this approach has essentially no role in the modern approach to the treatment of patients with advanced kidney cancer.

## 70. Is there a role for radiation therapy?

Radiation therapy has an effect on cancer by causing mutations to a cell's DNA, damaging it beyond repair. Cancer cells are generally more sensitive to radiation than healthy cells because they have already accumulated a number of mutations during malignant transformation. They are thus less likely to survive radiation. Certain cancer cells are more sensitive to radiation than others—this is a good treatment for some types of cancer (e.g., certain prostate cancers) but not for others. Another important principle is that radiation therapy to different parts of the body can cause a variety of side effects—the normal kidneys and small intestines are particularly sensitive to damage related to radiation therapy.

Kidney cancer cells are often resistant to radiation; thus this treatment is used only in special circumstances to treat metastatic kidney cancer. Such circumstances include tumors that cause pain (e.g., bone metastases), large tumors (e.g., a tumor obstructing the flow of air in the lung), or tumors in the brain. In these settings radiation therapy tends not to totally destroy the cancer, but it can shrink the cancer and relieve the symptoms. This can make a big difference for some patients even if it is only temporary.

Tumors in the brain can sometimes be removed surgically, but more often they are irradiated. Radiation to metastatic kidney cancer in the brain can either be whole brain radiation therapy (WBRT) or radiation focused just to the areas of tumor (called stereotactic radiosurgery or Gamma Knife radiation). This focused radiation can be very effective in controlling the areas that are irradiated, and allows the patient to avoid potentially disabling brain surgery. Whole brain radiation in particular can lead to slowing of the mental processes. In general, treatment of brain metastases must be undertaken prior to systemic therapy. The choice of what type of radiation to administer is made by the treating physicians in consultation with a specialist in radiation oncology.

## 71. Is there a role for vitamins and alternative treatments?

This is a difficult but common question, because patients like to play an active role in their care, and some patients are grasping at straws trying to avoid more aggressive treatments. The best way to think about vitamins or alternative treatments is that they may be complementary. They are unlikely to work by themselves, but when combined with proven effective treatments they may contribute to the final outcomes in a positive manner. Exactly how they do this and which alternative treatments are effective for kidney cancer is not known at this point in time.

One of the problems is that most vitamins and alternative therapies have not been tested in a rigorous manner—the FDA does not require this. Hence, we often do not have clear answers to many of the fundamental questions that are asked about these approaches, even the most basic ones: do their risks outweigh their benefits, and are they worth the cost?

It is important to stress that it would be naïve to think that there couldn't be potentially serious consequences to *anything* that one puts in one's body, whether it is a "natural" substance or not. Indeed there are well-documented instances of natural products interfering with anticancer therapies and/or producing toxicity that compromises the ability to deliver proven therapy. Common sense should prevail. That is, inform your doctor of everything you are doing outside of what he or she is prescribing so he/she can be aware of potential interactions and toxicity. Do not spend your life savings on promised miracle cures; there are plenty of people who will prey on your fears and insecurities and are happy to take your money for treatments that have plenty of testimonials but no real scientific support.

# PART EIGHT

# Immunotherapy

What is immunotherapy?

What is immunogenicity? How do we know
that kidney cancer is immunogenic?

What is interleukin-2 (IL-2)?

What are checkpoint control inhibitors?

*More*\*...

---

\*Words that may not be familiar to you are included in the glossary.
We have highlighted them in **bold** when they are first used in this book.

## 72. What is immunotherapy?

Immunotherapy is a general term for any anticancer therapy that attempts to kill cancer cells by "revving up the immune system." In so doing the immune system uses the same cells and processes that ordinarily fight off infection. All of the cells that make up the body's immune system work together as a unit (**Figure 22**). The body's immune system recognizes all of its own parts as "self" and anything else as "nonself." The body's immune system responds to anything that is "nonself," whether it is a splinter, an infection, or a cancer. The response consists of sending specialized immune cells and factors to the site of the intruder via the bloodstream.

Some of the major types of immune cells are dendritic cells (cells that process shredded pieces of infectious agents or cancers so that the immune system can mount a strong and specific response), B cells (lymphocytes that make antibodies to a foreign agent), and T cells (lymphocytes that coordinate and implement the cellular immune response). Antibodies produced by B cells stick to the foreign cells and are recognized by activated T cells that then come in for the kill. The immune system helps us fight off infection and cancer, usually but not always winning the battle. Some tumors are just too strong or have other defense mechanisms to evade the immune system, and these are the ones that we see in real life.

Many approaches to stimulate the body's immune system to fight off kidney cancer have been attempted in animals and people. The two most commonly used drugs have been interferon and interleukin-2 (IL-2). Although kidney cancer is considered a disease that can respond to this type of therapy, the percentage of patients who have any measurable response (tumor

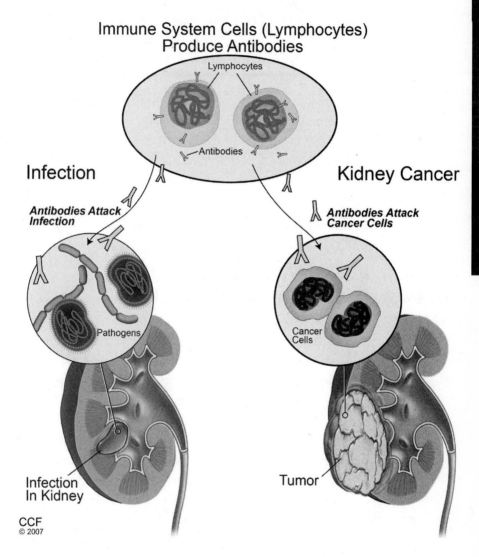

**Figure 22** The presence of infection with pathogens (bacteria, virus) within the kidney attracts immune cells to fight the infection. These include lymphocytes that make antibodies to the germs and target them for attack. The immune system also recognizes tumors since they often make proteins (antigens) that are not made by normal cells. The immune system is geared up to recognize foreign substances and to mount a response to eliminate them. In this way, our immune system allows us to fight infections and try to combat cancers like renal cell carcinoma.

shrinkage) to drugs like interferon and interleukin-2 is only 10–20%. So 80–90% of patients do not respond at all to the immunotherapy. Other experimental immunotherapy approaches (e.g., vaccines) have historically had limited clinical efficacy, although newer approaches are now being tested in clinical trials. Immunotherapy for kidney cancer is a concept with great potential, but for the most part this potential has not yet been realized.

## 73. What is immunogenicity? How do we know that kidney cancer is immunogenic?

**Immunogenicity**
The property of eliciting an immune response.

**Immunogenicity** means that the cancer is potentially sensitive to immunotherapy. There are three main reasons that kidney cancer is thought to be immunogenic. First, a very small number of patients (< 1%) with metastatic kidney cancer have tumors that disappear by themselves ("spontaneous regression"), suggesting that the body's immune system has eliminated the cancer cells. Second, a variety of scientific studies show infiltration of immune cells (lymphocytes) into kidney tumors, the expression of tumor-associated antigens, and the secretion of immune activating substances. All of these observations suggest that the body is mounting an immune response. Finally, and most importantly, patients with kidney cancer have been treated with immunotherapy for two to three decades and some of these patients have developed durable and complete responses. The 10–20% response rate to the immunotherapies interferon and interleukin indicates that kidney cancer is at least somewhat "immunogenic," and the occasional complete cures show that immunotherapy can work for this cancer. Unfortunately, only a minority of patients with metastatic kidney cancer responds to this approach.

## 74. What is interleukin-2 (IL-2)?

Interleukin-2 (IL-2) is a natural protein made by the body that normally helps to stimulate certain immune cells (called T cells) to fight off infections and cancer cells. It can be made in a laboratory and given through the vein or under the skin in an attempt to stimulate a patient's immune system to fight off the cancer. There are several ways to deliver IL-2 including "high-dose" IL-2, which is FDA-approved for the treatment of advanced kidney cancer, and "low-dose" IL-2, which is also occasionally used, but not FDA-approved. High-dose IL-2 is delivered through the vein three times each day in an ICU or similar closely monitored nursing care unit. This can shrink tumors in about 20% of patients (partial response) and, most importantly, a complete response and potential durable cure is observed in about 4–5% of patients (**Table 15**). This benefit is balanced against the toxicity of the treatment, which can cause very low blood pressure that can compromise the delivery of blood to all the major organs.

**Table 15**  Effect of Interleukin-2 and Interferon in Metastatic Kidney Cancer

|  | High-dose Interleukin-2 | Low-dose IL-2 or Interferon |
|---|---|---|
| Objective Response (tumors get at least 30% smaller) | 20% | 10–15% |
| Complete Response (tumors disappear) | 7–8% | 1–2% |
| Durable Complete Response (tumors disappear and never return) | 4–5% | rare |

High-dose IL-2 can therefore be very damaging to most of the body's working parts, including the heart, lungs, and kidneys. Typically, 14 doses of high-dose IL-2 are given over 5 days (if tolerated) and then repeated in 2 to 3 weeks, either until all tumors are gone, it is determined that the tumors are not responding to the treatment, or the patient can no longer tolerate the treatment. Most patients receive only a few rounds of treatment. Only healthy patients with clear cell kidney cancer can be considered for this intensive treatment modality. Low-dose IL-2 and low-dose interferon are currently rarely used in the treatment of metastatic renal cell carcinoma (RCC).

The reason for a patient to consider high-dose IL-2 is that it is the one treatment that is associated with a small, but real, chance of cure. The downsides to high-dose IL-2 are that the vast majority of patients (95%) will not be cured by this therapy and will still experience significant side effects. Because of the risks associated with treatment, high-dose IL-2 should be received only in a center with extensive experience in administration of this therapy. Most kidney cancer patients are not eligible to receive high-dose IL-2 because of advanced age, other health problems, or lack of access to centers with adequate expertise. Clear cell kidney cancers appear to respond best to IL-2, so IL-2 is now primarily reserved for patients with this type of kidney cancer. The role for IL-2 therapy is being redefined in the era of targeted therapy (see below).

Caregiver—Linda C.:

*Because Lori felt she had so much to live for she wanted to take the most aggressive treatment available and possibly get the one and only chance available for a cure. Other than the kidney cancer she was in good health and only age 32. She truly felt that the IL-2 treatments would be successful for her. She took her children's pictures and pinned them to the bulletin board across the room so she could be reminded WHY it was so important for her to take each treatment—and have the strength to continue on when the side effects were so severe.*

## 75. What is interferon?

Interferon alpha is also a natural protein that can be given as an injection under the skin to fight kidney cancer. Interferon normally functions to stimulate the immune system in many ways—it is another form of immunotherapy. Interferon is also known to have other mechanisms of action. It can kill cancer cells directly and it is also anti-angiogenic (inhibits blood vessels leading into the cancer and thus starves it of nutrients and oxygen). The relative importance of each of these anti-cancer effects is not well defined, but all are potentially beneficial. Interferon in kidney cancer is only given in relatively low doses under the skin and has similar benefits to low-dose IL-2 (Table 15). When compared to inactive treatments like hormonal therapy or chemotherapy, interferon was shown to make kidney cancer patients live longer, and it is for the most part a safe and tolerable therapy. Hence, interferon was considered a standard of care for many years. However, recent studies now show that the newer targeted therapies are more effective. Combining IL-2 and interferon can produce slightly higher tumor response rates, but has more side effects and does not extend life expectancy. Like low-dose IL-2, interferon is not approved by the FDA for the treatment of kidney cancer but is still occasionally used in this setting, particularly for patients who are not healthy enough to tolerate more aggressive treatments.

IMMUNOTHERAPY

## 76. *What other immunologic options are available, and what is inhibition of checkpoint control?*

As noted above, several experimental approaches to immunotherapy in kidney cancer are being investigated. These include interferon and IL-2-based approaches, vaccines, and other drugs that stimulate various immune cells. One of the more exciting new approaches is inhibition of a protein called programmed death ligand (PDL)-1 or its receptor (PD-1). Inhibition of these proteins through pharmacologic manipulation releases a natural "brake" on the immune system. This approach is now commonly referred to as "inhibition of checkpoint control." A similar approach has been to inhibit CTLA-4 expression on lymphocytes, which normally restrains the immune system. Again, inhibition of this factor allows the immune system to be reactivated. Preliminary clinical trials have shown safety and anti-tumor activity for these approaches. Many clinical trials of this approach either alone or in combination with targeted therapy are currently underway, and there is much excitement in the field about these trials. In addition, some new vaccine protocols (using a patient's tumor or a mixture of kidney cancer proteins injected under the skin) are in late stages of clinical testing.

# PART NINE

# *Targeted Molecular Therapy*

What is "targeted molecular" therapy?

How does Avastin® work?

How do Nexavar®, Sutent®, Votrient®, and Inlyta® work?

How do MTOR Inhibitors work?

*More*\*...

\*Words that may not be familiar to you are included in the glossary. We have highlighted them in **bold** when they are first used in this book.

## 77. What is "targeted molecular" therapy?

Targeted therapy is a general term in cancer medicine that means the drugs attack specific molecular targets that have been shown to be important in cancer cell growth. This specificity differentiates targeted therapy from traditional chemotherapy, which often indiscriminately kills any rapidly-dividing cell, including both cancer cells and some normal cells. The effects of chemotherapy on rapidly-dividing normal cells are responsible for many of the side effects of these treatments. For example, chemotherapy often causes damage to the cells that line the intestinal tract leading to gastrointestinal symptoms such as nausea, vomiting, and diarrhea. Another common adverse effect of chemotherapy is damage to the rapidly-dividing normal cells in the bone marrow leading to anemia, bleeding problems, and increased susceptibility to infection.

In theory, targeted therapy should kill cancer cells while sparing normal cells from damage, thus avoiding side effects. In reality, targeted therapy can be limited by several factors. First, the molecular target of a specific agent may also function in some normal cellular processes. These processes can be disrupted by targeted therapy. For example, VEGF, one of the major proteins that stimulates tumor angiogenesis (growth of new blood vessels that feed a tumor), also plays an active role in normal wound healing, so agents that target this molecular pathway might also cause delayed wound healing. Targeted molecular therapy is often not specific against just one target and can have side effects related to blocking other targets. Additionally, therapy that attacks just one target may not be enough to kill all of the cancer cells or to do so permanently. Targeted therapy may be best used as just one component of an integrated treatment plan for advanced cancer.

Truly targeted therapy that affects only cancer cells and does not interfere with normal cells (thus no side effects) is not yet available at this point in time. However, the new targeted therapies are still a major step forward, because their side effects appear to be much more manageable than those of chemotherapy and they have shown impressive activity against some cancers that often do not respond to chemotherapy. Kidney cancer is one of these cancers.

## 78. How does Avastin® work?

Avastin (bevacizumab) has been approved by the United States Food and Drug Administration (FDA) for metastatic colon and lung cancer, and is now also approved for metastatic kidney cancer when used along with interferon. Most of the new molecular treatments for kidney cancer target VEGF (**Figure 23**), also known as vascular endothelial growth factor (see Question 13 for additional details about VEGF). VEGF is the main factor made by kidney cancers that stimulates angiogenesis and tumor growth. Kidney cancer cells secrete VEGF and this causes a sprouting of blood vessels into the tumor. The tumor needs these blood vessels to supply itself with oxygen and nutrients for accelerated tumor growth. The tumor also can take advantage of the blood vessels to invade them and get into the bloodstream and metastasize to other parts of the body. Blocking angiogenesis has been one of the main goals of targeted molecular treatments in this era.

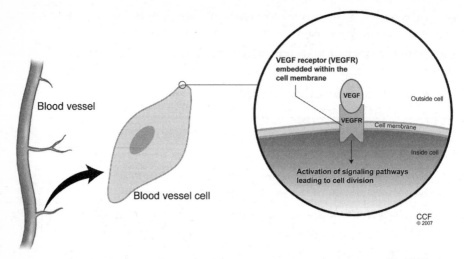

**Figure 23** Targeted molecular agents act by blocking the growth of new blood vessels. A growth factor released by tumor cells, VEGF, binds to a receptor present on the surface of blood vessel cells. The binding of VEGF to its receptor (VEGFR) leads to activation of several pathways within the cell that cause the blood vessel cells to divide and sprout to form new blood vessels. These blood vessels provide oxygen and nutrients to the growing tumor.

Reprinted with permission, Cleveland Clinic Center for Medical Art & Photography © 2007–2014. All Rights Reserved.

Avastin is an antibody produced in the laboratory that binds to VEGF (**Figure 24**). Avastin is given through the vein (intravenously, or IV). When it binds to VEGF it sequesters it so that the VEGF is no longer active. Angiogenesis is turned off and the tumor vessels can retract—this leads to a starving of the tumor. Overall, Avastin leads to tumor shrinkage in most patients, some just a small amount and some more dramatically. Most impressively, Avastin has been shown to slow the progression of kidney cancer in a trial that compared its effects when combined with interferon versus a placebo

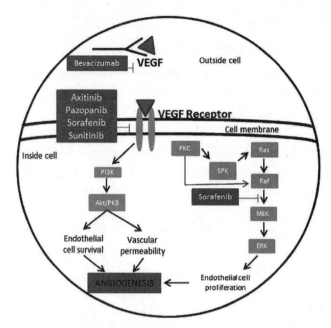

**Figure 24** The VEGF pathway plays an important role in kidney cancer. The mechanisms of action of Avastin and TKIs are shown. Avastin (bevacizumab) binds and sequesters VEGF and the TKI's block the receptor for VEGF.

Reprinted with permission, Cleveland Clinic Center for Medical Art & Photography © 2007–2014. All Rights Reserved.

infusion combined with interferon. Avastin is now considered one of the VEGF-targeted treatments for patients with advanced kidney cancer.

Caregiver—Linda C.:

*Avastin was the only treatment that gave Lori positive results. Avastin did not "shrink" Lori's tumors, but it did give her more than 6 months of stability, which in turn gave her more time and memories with and for her children. She had many good days during the year she took the Avastin and we will always be grateful for each moment.*

## 79. How do Nexavar®, Sutent®, Votrient®, and Inlyta® work?

All of these drugs are oral pills that inhibit VEGF in a different way than Avastin. They are a class of drugs known as small molecule tyrosine kinase inhibitors (TKIs). For VEGF to work it must bind to a protein (called the VEGF receptor) that is present on the surface of blood vessel cells (endothelial cells). When VEGF binds to its receptor, this triggers a cascade of events that leads to angiogenesis. During this process downstream molecular pathways are activated and the endothelial cell begins to divide and to form new blood vessels. TKIs such as Nexavar (sorafenib), Sutent (sunitinib), and the others block this pathway by inactivating the VEGF receptor so that it can no longer respond to VEGF, and angiogenesis is inhibited (**Figure 25**).

TKIs promote tumor shrinkage in many patients, and stability in others. Tumor stability means that the tumor does not grow and this is a good thing—if it would stay this way forever, the patient would not suffer any ill effects from the tumor. Unfortunately, the tumor eventually becomes resistant to the effects of a given TKI and will begin to grow. But in the meantime the progressive effects of the cancer have been slowed, and this will often buy the patient several good months (and sometimes even longer) before tumor progression occurs. A total cure is rarely seen and this is typical for this class of drugs—they tend to be tumoristatic (slow the growth of the tumor) rather than tumoricidal (directly and completely kill the cancer cells).

Sutent and Votrient (pazopanib) are somewhat different than the other targeted agents in that they appear to

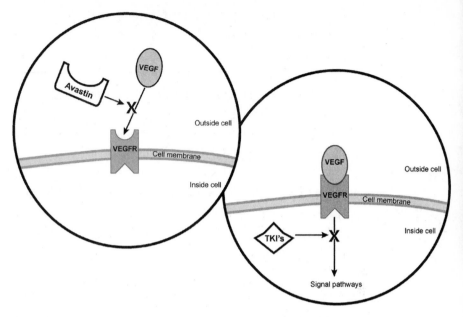

**Figure 25** Avastin binds and sequesters VEGF making it inoperative while TIKs inhibit the receptor of VEGF and block downstream pathways.

Reprinted with permission, Cleveland Clinic Center for Medical Art & Photography
© 2007–2014. All Rights Reserved.

have the ability to shrink tumors more dramatically, and thus may have advantages for patients with symptomatic and/or large tumors.

Sutent is one of the more commonly used agents. It has been shown to delay the progression of kidney cancer more effectively than treatment with interferon in kidney cancer patients. Patients taking Sutent are given one pill daily for 28 days, followed by 14 days of rest, after which this 6-week cycle is repeated. Again, a total cure is not common, but tumor shrinkage and delay of tumor progression are often achieved, representing major gains for most patients with advanced kidney cancer. Other TKIs provide similar benefits and all are taken orally.

Votrient is another TKI that acts against the VEGF receptor. It was shown to delay disease progression compared to placebo in a trial. This drug is taken once per day on an empty stomach. A recent trial showed it had similar effectiveness as Sutent. The side effect profiles, however, are different between these two drugs (and among all the TKIs); thus your doctor may prefer one TKI over another due to a more favorable side effect profile for you.

Inlyta (axitinib) is the newest TKI that showed delayed disease progression compared to Nexavar in patients who had already been on one therapy such as Sutent or IL-2. This drug is now being tested in untreated patients.

Patient—Dennis W.:

*After being on IL-2, and thalidomide, interferon, and Sutent®, I can tell you that there are good sides and bad sides to each. However, Sutent® had a much more subtle set of side effects for me than the other two. They are no less disturbing, but just different. The fatigue with Sutent® is hard to describe. With this drug, when fatigue set in for me, it was immediate and complete. It was not like hitting the wall, then recouping, and then going again. With this, when I hit the wall, I was spent. I am sure it is different for every individual.*

## 80. How do Torisel® and Afinitor® work?

Torisel (temsirolimus) and Afinitor (everolimus) work by inhibiting a protein called mTOR (mammalian target of rapamycin). This protein is part of an intracellular pathway that may have effects on both cancer cell proliferation and VEGF production. These drugs inhibit the kinase activity of mTOR, which regulates the cell's protein-making machinery and is central to cell growth (see **Figure 26**). When this pathway is blocked, the cell is halted at a specific phase of the cell cycle and stops dividing.

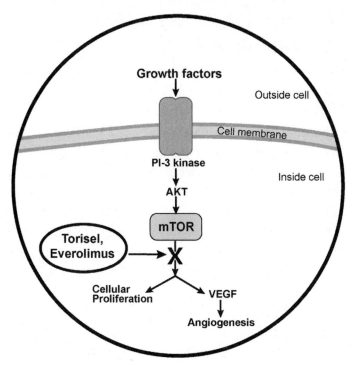

**Figure 26** Mechanism of action of mTOR inhibitors. Torisel® (temsirolimus) and Afinitor® (everolimus) block the mTOR protein and thus block the downstream pathways that are important for tumor progression.

Torisel was FDA-approved in May 2007 and has been shown to prolong life in kidney cancer patients with disease features that generally predict a poor outcome. This group of patients has been notoriously difficult to treat, but Torisel was able to prolong survival. Torisel provides significantly higher median overall survival and progression-free survival compared with interferon-alpha (IFN-a).

Afinitor has been shown to delay disease progression compared to placebo in kidney cancer patients who have received two or more prior treatments. This drug is taken as a daily pill.

## 81. How were the targeted molecular agents developed?

The story begins with a series of careful scientific observations that led to the identification of VEGF as a key molecule in angiogenesis and the identification and sequencing of the VEGF protein and its receptors. Then the pharmaceutical companies synthesized hundreds and in some cases thousands of small molecules that could potentially block the receptors—each molecule was designed to fit the receptor domain in an effort to mimic the active part of VEGF, with each molecule being slightly different due to various side groups and other modifications. Each of these molecules had to be tested in the laboratory to see which one would block the VEGF receptor most effectively, and the best candidates were then moved forward to testing in animals. The animal studies were performed to see which of these candidates would work best in a live situation, and to make sure that the drugs were safe and tolerable. The drugs were then moved into human trials. As you can imagine, this whole process was very expensive, often costing several hundreds of millions of dollars to safely evaluate and develop a drug that could be used in cancer patients.

*Targeted molecular agents are generally very active against kidney cancer when compared to treatments that have been used in the past.*

The second half of the story deals with the drug after it has been developed in the laboratory. All of the targeted molecular therapies were developed through clinical trials conducted in patients with metastatic kidney cancer. The details of each trial are somewhat different, but the goals of these trials are first to demonstrate the agent's safety and later its efficacy. Some of these trials required patients to get a placebo pill before later being treated with active drug. Other trials randomized patients to receive either a placebo pill or the agent being evaluated; neither the patient nor the treating physician knows what any individual patient is receiving—we say that they are blinded. Although placebo trials are not desirable to patients or physicians, they are often required in order to most clearly see a drug's benefit and ultimately lead to FDA approval so that more kidney cancer patients can benefit. Cancer progression while on a clinical trial often results in the removal of the patient from the trial so that they can receive some other type of treatment. When an agent is shown to have a definite benefit in the context of a clinical trial, most trials allow patients who had been receiving placebo to switch over to receive the active agent. Importantly, ongoing clinical trials of these and other drugs are required to extend the benefits of these agents. Clinical trials are critically important to advance our knowledge and move the field forward for the benefit of all kidney cancer patients.

## 82. Do these new targeted molecular agents work and which is best for me?

Targeted molecular agents are generally very active against kidney cancer when compared to treatments that have been used in the past. Activity against cancer may mean that the drug is able to cause the tumors to get smaller by a little or a lot, delay the progression of disease, or even prolong life. It is not presently possible to predict whether a specific patient will benefit from a specific drug or drugs. Therefore, your doctor will need to choose your therapy based on factors such as side effect profile, ease of administration, characteristics of your kidney cancer, and prior treatments. Clinical trials have not been able to compare all active targeted agents against each other, so it is not presently possible to say which new agent is "best." Advanced kidney cancer remains difficult to treat, and even when a beneficial effect is seen with one agent, the cancer may progress at some point in time. It is therefore likely that most kidney cancer patients will receive more than one of these therapies during the course of their disease. But the long and short of this answer is that the new targeted agents do work for most patients, either leading to tumor shrinkage or stability, and typically delaying progression of their disease. These agents are more effective than chemotherapy or immunotherapy and are considered state-of-the-art treatment for most patients with advanced kidney cancer.

## 83. What is the likelihood of a cure with targeted molecular agents?

Doctors have only recently started treating patients with these agents; there is therefore not a large population of patients who have been treated for more than a few years. In general, most patients treated with targeted molecular therapy do not have complete disappearance of tumors, and thus cannot be considered cured. However, these agents can control the spread of disease for many months to years, and it is possible that the drugs may be able to cause the tumors to shrink enough to have them surgically removed, and thus possibly be cured. Further experience will be required to determine the actual cure rate with these agents.

*Patients with advanced kidney cancer should speak with physicians knowledgeable about kidney cancer to decide which treatment option is best for them.*

## 84. Should I have high-dose IL-2 or targeted molecular therapy?

This is a difficult and complicated question, and there is no clear answer. Here are the main considerations:

- High dose IL-2 is the only treatment for advanced kidney cancer that has been shown in clinical trials to have a small but real chance (4–5%) of cure. This benefit is offset by the fact that only a select group of patients is eligible to receive it and fit enough to tolerate the toxicity of treatment. The treatment can be very rigorous and can be associated with substantial morbidity and a very small but finite risk of death.

- Targeted therapies are more recently introduced and not known to produce a durable complete response, so a total cure is unlikely. On the other hand, these treatments do delay the rate of cancer progression. Clinical trials have shown that they are superior to immunotherapy in this regard and exhibit less toxicity. They are taken orally, or intravenously (IV), and are associated with fewer side effects, and the side effects appear to be less severe than those associated with high-dose IL-2.

Patients with advanced kidney cancer should gather all available information and speak with physicians knowledgeable about kidney cancer to decide which treatment option is best for them. In reality, most kidney cancer patients will ultimately end up receiving several treatments, and thus the question is not which agent to choose, but in what order the various therapeutic options should be pursued.

## 85. What are the side effects of targeted molecular agents?

Targeted molecular therapies, like all anticancer therapies, have side effects. The side effects are likely to be different for each person in terms of which specific side effects will occur, the severity of the symptoms, and their timing of onset and/or resolution. One theoretical concern with all of these agents is that they may inhibit wound healing, and this could be a major concern if the patient required surgery or was in an accident. However, to date, this has not been found to be a common or substantial problem with these drugs. In addition, all agents that affect VEGF (and thus are affecting blood vessels) have the potential to cause bleeding or lead to the formation of blood clots. The likelihood of bleeding and/or forming blood clots, however, appears to be relatively low (around 1–2%).

- Avastin is generally well tolerated by patients on a day-to-day basis. Major side effects include high blood pressure and spillage of protein into the urine. Avastin has also very rarely caused perforation (a hole) in the intestines, a potentially serious condition, for unknown reasons.

- TKIs have additional side effects including fatigue, diarrhea, soreness of the mouth, and soreness of the palms and soles of the feet (called hand/foot syndrome). These drugs can also raise blood pressure. Sutent can also affect the thyroid gland and thus some patients may require a thyroid replacement hormone pill (called Synthroid) while on Sutent. Your doctor should check thyroid function blood tests before and during Sutent administration.

- Torisel and Afinitor can cause elevation of blood sugar and triglycerides. They can also rarely cause inflammation of the lungs, which can lead to shortness of breath. The most common (incidence $\geq 30\%$) adverse reactions observed with Torisel are rash, asthenia, mucositis, nausea, edema, and anorexia.

It is important to note that, because the targeted agents are still relatively new, not all of their potential side effects are known. There may be rare but serious side effects, as well as those associated with long-term use, which have not yet been determined. If you are taking one of these medications it is vital that you inform your doctor immediately of any side effects you may be experiencing.

## 86. How is hypertension caused by targeted agents treated and what does it signify?

All patients on targeted therapy should undergo regular monitoring of their blood pressure, because the development of hypertension or exacerbation of already existing hypertension is a common side effect of these medications. If the blood pressure is increasing on targeted therapy, the patient may need to be started on antihypertensive medications, or have additional antihypertensive medications added or doses increased. If this fails, the dose of the targeted agent may need to be decreased, or a different targeted agent may need to be considered. Most oncologists feel strongly that it is important to try to make adjustments to keep the patient on the current therapy if possible, because dose reductions or changes in therapy can often prove to be counterproductive. Stated in a simpler manner, if the patient is responding to a given targeted agent, it is best to keep him/her on this agent and dose if possible.

One interesting observation is that patients who develop hypertension on therapy appear to respond better to the treatment—at least this appears to be the case with Sutent. It is not yet known if this will prove to be true with the other targeted agents. It is important to emphasize that the corollary is not necessarily true, and patients should not undergo dose acceleration in an effort to stimulate hypertension.

## 87. What is hand-foot syndrome?

Hand-foot syndrome is a term used to describe the redness, soreness, and blistering that can sometimes occur with TKIs such as Sutent and Nexavar. It occurs in approximately 30–50% of patients and tends to be worse on areas that are subjected to pressure. The causes of hand-foot syndrome are not currently known. The severity of these symptoms can vary; some patients have a little redness, but others can experience significant discomfort. The appearances of a mild and a more severe case are demonstrated in **Figure 27**. If pain occurs, it is generally required that the patient stop the Sutent or Nexavar to allow time for this to resolve. This side effect can be severe or disabling in 5–10% of patients and can lead to a reduction in dose or even discontinuation of the medicine. Topical agents, such as creams, can be used to manage the symptoms.

## 88. How long should I be treated with a targeted molecular agent and how will I be followed?

It is unclear how long treatment with these new agents should last. In general, many patients have some but not complete tumor shrinkage, and thus are treated continuously until the disease worsens or side effects become too severe. It is not clear that this strategy is optimal, and long-term therapy with these agents may lead to side effects that can substantially affect quality of life. Strategies to give therapy intermittently are being considered but are not yet proven.

As you proceed with therapy, follow-up CT scans and other relevant imaging studies and laboratory tests will

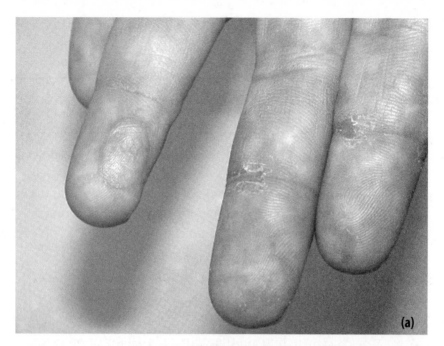

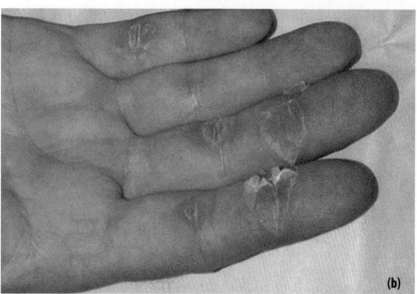

**Figure 27** Hand-foot syndrome can be mild (a) or severe (b). This side effect of targeted molecular therapy leads to blistering and ulceration of the skin, typically on the hands and feet. Symptoms typically resolve if treatment is discontinued temporarily or permanently.

be obtained to monitor your progress. Your doctor will ask you about side effects. This can lead to a number of different outcomes:

- Treatment with the same drug will continue if there has been stabilization or shrinkage of the tumor and you are tolerating the treatment well.

- Surgery may be considered if the tumor sites have shrunk substantially and are now limited in their involvement to the point that total surgical excision might be possible. Unfortunately, only a minority of patients will fall into this group.

- Observation may be appropriate if the tumor is stable and you need a break from therapy due to side effects or other considerations—sometimes patients just need a break from active treatment.

- A switch to another targeted therapy or other systemic agent may be required, particularly if there is progression of disease—a clinical trial should always be considered in this instance.

- A palliative course of action (comfort as first priority) may need to be considered if the tumor is rapidly progressive and not responding to other available therapies.

Each patient should be managed on an individual basis taking all of these factors into consideration. Good communication with your physician can help to optimize these important decision-making processes.

## 89. Can one agent work when another has failed?

The new targeted molecular agents were first studied in patients who had disease that had progressed despite immunotherapy using IL-2 or interferon. Subsequent studies have shown clear activity of one targeted agent after another has failed, although usually with less activity for the second targeted agent when compared to a first. The optimal sequence for the use of these agents is not yet defined. In reality, your doctor is likely to try a sequence of several of the targeted agents during the course of your disease.

## 90. Do I need to start targeted therapy immediately and do I need to be on it continuously?

When first diagnosed with metastatic disease you may be asymptomatic and have a relatively low burden of disease, e.g., just a few small lung metastases. In this setting the cancer may be somewhat indolent, and a trial of observation without active therapy should be considered. With this pathway you can be monitored with CT scans and other studies, and therapy can be initiated when substantial progression is observed, or if you begin to develop symptoms.

Regarding whether you need to be on therapy continuously, the answer is that intermittent therapy can often be considered. As mentioned in Question 88, for many patients it is helpful to take a break from therapy to get relief from the chronic side effects of therapy, such as fatigue. During the break from therapy you can be monitored and therapy can be restarted if there is evidence of substantial tumor progression.

## 91. Will combinations of targeted agents work better than single agents?

It makes sense that when there is more than one active treatment against a certain type of cancer to consider combining these treatments either at the same time or one after the other (sequentially). However, combinations of the various targeted agents have proven in general too toxic and no more effective than single agents. Newer combinations are being tested in clinical trials, but to date no combination (outside of Avastin combined with interferon) should be used outside of a trial.

## 92. Is there still a role for nephrectomy in patients receiving targeted molecular therapy?

The short answer is *yes*. Nephrectomy in properly-selected patients has been shown to make patients with metastatic kidney cancer live longer (see Question 66). In these trials the patients received interferon after nephrectomy rather than targeted therapy, so it is not clearly established that nephrectomy will also benefit patients who will subsequently receive targeted therapies. However, there is still very good reason to believe that surgery is of benefit for patients who will receive agents other than interferon, and this is the standard of care that is currently practiced in this era.

Still, the optimal timing of nephrectomy relative to treatment with a targeted therapy is currently unknown. The role of targeted agents in shrinking large primary tumors to make surgery safer or more effective is not yet known— this is an active area of investigation. Importantly, nephrectomy is not recommended for all patients with metastatic kidney cancer. The best candidates are those who are otherwise healthy, who have the majority of the overall tumor burden in the kidney, and in whom surgery is able to safely remove the kidney. Patients who do not meet these criteria should receive systemic therapy first and then be reassessed for surgery later.

## 93. Can I have surgery later to "clean things up?"

The short answer here is *maybe but probably not*. Given that the new agents can shrink tumors, it is possible that surgery could be done after a response has been obtained with targeted therapy. This should be considered only if the doctors can be reasonably sure that surgery will remove all of the visible cancer that remains. To put it another way, given the risks of surgery in this setting, it should be considered only if there is a chance that it might lead to a cure. Yet, even in the best of circumstances, there is a real risk that the cancer will return—the cancer that is evident and resected may be only the "tip of the iceberg." The best candidates for this aggressive approach are those who are relatively healthy and those with only limited sites of disease located in surgically amenable sites.

Another important consideration is that the risks of surgery may be increased in patients taking targeted therapies because of potential effects on the blood vessels (possibly increased risks of surgical bleeding or clot formation) and negative effects on wound healing. The safety of surgery in this setting appears to be reasonable, but is still being investigated. In addition, there are no firm guidelines as to how long a patient should be off therapy before or after surgery to facilitate safe surgery and good outcomes.

## 94. What new agents are on the horizon?

Metastatic kidney cancer has entered a new era of treatment where drugs targeting specific proteins are making a big impact in this disease. Additional proteins and other targets will emerge in the near future, all driven by important research advances, and thus new agents to attack these targets will be tested in clinical trials. Continued laboratory research and clinical trials will be essential to move this field forward. Recent protocols using immunotherapy hold much promise and studies utilizing these approaches should be supported whenever feasible.

# PART TEN

# Clinical Trials

What is a clinical trial?

What is informed consent?

How do I know that someone is making
sure that the clinical trials are conducted
in a safe and ethical manner?

*More*[*]...

*[*]Words that may not be familiar to you are included in the glossary.
We have highlighted them in **bold** when they are first used in this book.

## 95. What is a clinical trial?

Clinical trials are research studies using human volunteers (also called participants) that are intended to add to medical knowledge. A clinical trial is a formal evaluation of the safety and effectiveness of a given drug or therapeutic protocol. Before a drug is given to patients, it generally has been tested extensively in the laboratory and in animals and found to have some effect.

Clinical trials are led by a *principal investigator*, who is often a medical doctor. There is typically a research team that includes doctors, nurses, social workers, and other healthcare professionals. A clinical trial is conducted according to a research plan known as the protocol. The *protocol* is designed to answer specific research questions as well as safeguard the health of participants.

Participants in a clinical trial receive specific interventions, which may be medical products, such as drugs or devices; procedures (e.g., changes in the way a given treatment is done); or changes to participants' behavior, for example, a new diet. Clinical trials may compare a new medical approach to a standard one that is already available or to a placebo (a substance having no effect but administered as a control in testing). The investigators try to determine the safety and efficacy of the intervention by measuring certain outcomes in the participants. Clinical trials used in drug development are sometimes described by phase. These phases are defined by the Food and Drug Administration (FDA).

Clinical testing in patients can include:
- Phase I: The earliest trials of a drug in humans are designed to determine the safe dose of the drug and the frequency of administration. These trials

are called phase I trials. Participants on phase I trials have already received standard treatment for their specific cancer and have progressed or are no longer able to tolerate this treatment. Many of these patients have run out of options and need to consider new drugs for treatment. Different doses of the new drug(s) are given to various patients to determine the safe dose level.

- Phase II: After determining a safe dosing schedule for a given drug in phase I trials, the next step is a phase II trial. These trials take the safe dose regimen from the phase I trials and apply them to a small (approximately 30–50) patient population, usually all with a single disease like kidney cancer. These trials are done to further define the safety of the drug, and also to begin to find out if the drug has any antitumor activity, as measured in tumor shrinkage or duration of time until tumors grow.

- Phase III: Agents that show activity in phase II trials are then evaluated in a phase III trial, which compares a *new therapy* to the *standard treatment* in a given disease circumstance. This allows for a direct comparison to see if the new therapy is a step forward compared to standard treatment.

Completion of a large phase III trial (usually 600–900 patients) is generally required for a drug to be approved by the FDA. Often additional studies (sometimes called phase IV or postmarketing studies) are done after FDA approval to study the drug in additional patients and/or in different disease circumstances. Clinical trial participation is vital for us to improve cancer care.

While most clinical trials provide participants with medical products or interventions related to the illness or condition being studied, they do not usually provide extended or complete health care. Clinical trial participants often continue to see their usual healthcare providers. By having the patient's usual healthcare provider work with the research team, the patient can make sure that the study protocol will not conflict with other medications or treatments being received.

## 96. What is informed consent?

Informed consent is a process in which researchers provide potential participants with information about a clinical study. Informed consent means that before a patient goes on any type of clinical trial, he or she needs to be well informed about the potential risks, benefits, and alternatives to the specific therapy. This involves a 10–15 page document that carefully spells out in simple language the good and bad features of a drug or approach and lets patients know the other treatment options. This information helps patients decide whether they want to enroll, or continue to participate, in the study. The informed consent process is intended to protect participants and should provide enough information for a person to understand the risks, potential benefits, and alternatives to the study.

Informed consent does not mean there are not very real risks to the treatment being studied, only that a patient is informed of these risks before being treated. If you are considered for a clinical trial you should take the time to read the description of the trial and make sure that you understand all of the options and risks involved. Do not hesitate to ask questions.

## 97. How do I know that someone is making sure that the clinical trials are conducted in a safe and ethical manner?

Each federally supported or conducted clinical study and each study of a drug, biological product, or medical device regulated by the FDA must be reviewed, approved, and monitored by an institutional review board (IRB). The IRB is comprised of scientific experts, legal advisors, and patient advocates who review and approve all research protocols and consent forms before patients are allowed to sign them and participate in the clinical trials. Its role is to make sure that the study is ethical and the rights and welfare of participants are protected. This includes making sure that research risks are minimized and are reasonable in relation to any potential benefits, among other things.

The IRB takes great pains to make sure that all research is conducted in a safe and fair manner, and all institutional IRBs are monitored regularly to make sure that they are following all appropriate guidelines. Multiple levels of regulation are involved and all strive to protect the safety and autonomy of patients.

## 98. How do I decide whether I should participate in a clinical trial?

Participation in clinical trials is the only way that new and better drugs for kidney cancer or any disease can be discovered. You should carefully weigh all available information about a given clinical trial and all reasonable treatment alternatives before deciding to participate. In the end, you must be comfortable with your treating physician and treatment approach before undertaking any treatment, including treatment on a clinical trial.

Patients interested in participating in a clinical trial should learn as much as they can about the study and should feel comfortable asking the research team questions. The National Institutes of Health suggests a few questions on their website *www.ClinicalTrials.gov*. Some of the answers are found in the informed consent documents. Suggested questions to ask include:

- What is being studied?
- Why do researchers believe the intervention being tested might be effective? Why might it not be effective? Has it been tested before?
- What are the possible interventions that I might receive during the trial?
- How will it be determined which interventions I receive (for example, by chance)?
- Who will know which intervention I receive during the trial? Will I know? Will members of the research team know?
- How do the possible risks, side effects, and benefits of this trial compare with those of my current treatment?
- What will I have to do?
- What tests and procedures are involved?
- How often will I have to visit the hospital or clinic?
- Will hospitalization be required?
- How long will the study last?
- Who will pay for my participation?
- Will I be reimbursed for other expenses?
- What type of long-term follow-up care is part of this trial?

- If I benefit from the intervention, will I be allowed to continue receiving it after the trial ends?
- Will results of the study be provided to me?
- Who will oversee my medical care while I am in the trial?
- What are my options if I am injured during the study?

Caregiver—Linda C.:

*If there are no FDA-approved drugs that have proven to be effective for your loved one, I believe the patient and the family should research all the clinical trials available to them. After doing this they should discuss these options with their RCC specialist or oncologist. Knowledge is power. The more knowledge the patient has regarding this disease, the better his or her chance for survival.*

*It is imperative for both the patient AND the family/care-givers to be proactive in the treatments available. The patient is already going through so much with treatments, it is so very important that family members educate themselves FOR their loved one.*

*There are so many different kinds of cancers, there are so many different types of treatments—a doctor is only human—he cannot possibly know EVERYTHING. I think we should help in whatever way we can and educate our-selves in whatever way possible.*

*The IRB takes great pains to make sure that all research is conducted in a safe and fair manner. Participation in clinical trials is the only way that new and better drugs for kidney cancer or any cancer can be discovered.*

## 99. How can I learn more about clinical trials?

There are two key sources of information about clinical trials. The National Cancer Institute (NCI) and the National Institutes of Health (NIH) both offer additional information about clinical trials, as well as listings of current, recent, and future studies.

The website *www.ClinicalTrials.gov*, a service of the NIH, is the National Library of Medicine-developed web-based registry and results database of clinical research studies. The website provides patients, clinicians, researchers, and the public with access to information about interventional and observational studies.

You may call the Cancer Information Service (CIS) at: 1-800-4-CANCER (1-800-422-6237) or TTY: 1-800-332-8615, or visit the NCI website: *http://cancertrials.nci.nih.gov*. The NCI has a comprehensive database about cancer and clinical trials called Physician Data Query (PDQ). The PDQ is regularly updated and supplies information on more than 4,000 clinical trials worldwide, as well as contacts for the physicians and institutions conducting the trials. Treatment studies are grouped by disease site, treatment type, study phase, study drug, and study location. Supportive care studies are grouped by the cancer-related problem (for example, pain, anemia, infection), while prevention/ early detection studies are grouped by cancer type. Patients can obtain PDQ information from their physicians or by contacting the CIS. Your doctor should also be able to provide additional information. It is important to realize that the results of a given trial are not available until many months or longer after the trial is fully completed. Therefore, you will not be able to decide about your participation in a trial based on known results, but rather potential benefits weighed against known side effects.

Caregiver—Linda C.:

*Have family members get involved and do research. The Internet can be very helpful with this. But be careful and check with your physician because there is questionable information out there. All of the treatments on the Internet may not apply to you. Many sell false hope. Remember "knowledge is power." The more knowledge you have, the better your chance for survival. Be proactive in your treatments!*

## 100. How can I learn more about kidney cancer?

There are several sources of information. Your doctor and/or a doctor who specializes in kidney cancer are ultimately the best sources because they know all of the particulars of your situation. Several Internet sites may also have useful information.

The Urology Care Foundation, the official foundation of the American Urological Association, is a nonprofit organization whose goal is to promote health, provide hope, and promise a future free of urological disease, including cancer. You can reach the Urology Care Foundation at 1-800-828-7866 or visit their website, *www.UrologyHealth.org*, for information on kidney cancer and various treatment options.

The Kidney Cancer Association (KCA) is a national kidney cancer group that is an outstanding resource. They provide patient literature and conduct conferences and support groups to educate kidney cancer patients.

The KCA can be reached at 1-800-850-9132 or by visiting their website, *www.KidneyCancer.org*.

Contacting other kidney cancer patients who have undergone similar experiences can also be helpful. You can ask your doctor if there are other patients who may be willing to discuss their experience with you.

The National Cancer Institute (NCI) is a component of the National Institutes of Health (NIH), one of eight agencies that compose the Public Health Service (PHS) in the Department of Health and Human Services (DHHS). The National Cancer Institute coordinates the National Cancer Program, which conducts and supports research, training, health information dissemination, and other programs with respect to the cause, diagnosis, prevention, and treatment of cancer, rehabilitation from cancer, and the continuing care of cancer patients and the families of cancer patients. You can access NCI information about kidney cancer online at *www.Cancer.gov*.

# *Glossary*

## A

**Abdomen**: The cavity of the body containing the stomach, intestines, liver, and spleen. The kidneys are located behind this cavity.

**Active surveillance**: Active surveillance is also known as watchful waiting or observation which simply means that a physician and a patient work together to actively observe an identified renal mass. Radiographic tests such as a CT scan, MRI scan, or ultrasound are done at regular intervals to observe the mass.

**Adjuvant treatment**: Utilizing medications, radiation therapy, or other means of supplemental treatment following cancer surgery.

**Adrenal glands**: A small gland located on top of the kidney. The adrenal glands produce hormones that help control heart rate, blood pressure, the way the body uses food, the levels of minerals such as sodium and potassium in the blood, and other functions particularly involved in stress reactions.

**Adrenaline**: A hormone secreted by the adrenal glands that helps the body meet the demands of physical or emotional stress.

**Allele**: Any of the possible forms in which a gene for a specific trait can occur.

**Analogous**: Having similar function but a different structure and origin.

**Anechoic**: Not having or producing echoes. Used to describe solid lesions on ultrasound, because they do not send back echoes.

**Angiogenesis**: The formation of new blood vessels, especially blood vessels that supply oxygen and nutrients to cancerous tissues.

**Angiomyolipoma**: A benign tumor composed of fat tissue, muscle cells, and vascular structures.

**Anti-angiogenic treatment**: Medication that prevents cancer growth by limiting the growth of new blood vessels that provide nutrients for cancer expansion.

**Antibodies**: Proteins in the blood that are produced by the body in response to specific foreign proteins (such as bacteria). Antibodies then trigger the immune system to respond to the foreign proteins.

**Apoptosis**: Process by which a cell eliminates itself, also known as programmed cell death. The body uses this process to delete cells that have acquired mutations that may cause them to become cancerous.

**Arteries**: Blood vessels that carry blood to an organ, such as the kidney.

**Autosomal dominant**: A pattern of inheritance in which half of the offspring will receive the mutated gene and develop the syndrome possessed by the parent.

**B**

**Benign**: Of no danger to health; not recurrent or progressive; not malignant: a benign tumor.

**Bland thrombus**: A blood clot inside of a vein. This is in contrast to the growth of tumor cells within the vein, that can occur in kidney cancer paients

**Bowels**: The intestines.

**C**

**Cancer**: An uncontrolled growth of cells.

**Carcinogen**: Any substance or agent that tends to produce a cancer.

**Carcinoma**: An invasive malignant tumor derived from epithelial tissue that tends to metastasize to other areas of the body.

**Cell**: The smallest unit of life that is classified as a living thing. Each cell contains all of the basic structural and functional components of living organisms, also known as the building blocks of life.

**Chemotherapy**: The treatment of cancer using specific chemical agents or drugs that are selectively destructive to malignant cells and tissues.

**Chromophobe renal cell carcinoma**: An uncommon type of kidney cancer responsible for less than 5% of kidney cancers. Most of these tumors do not spread outside of the kidney.

**Chromosome**: All of a person's genes (genome) are encoded on 23 pairs of chromosomes. Each chromosome consists of two intertwined strands of DNA wrapped around a protein core.

**Clear cell renal cell carcinoma**: Most common type of kidney cancer, representing 70–80% of all cases of renal cell carcinoma, generally characterized by cells with clear cytoplasm. Genetic event responsible for this subtype is mutation or inactivation of the VHL gene on chromosome 3.

**Creatinine**: A breakdown product of muscle that is filtered by the kidney and measured in the blood or urine. Measurement in the blood or urine can provide an estimate of kidney function.

**Cryoablation**: Refers to destruction of a tumor by superfreezing. This procedure can be performed either under laparoscopic guidance or sometimes with radiographic guidance without the need for surgery. Also known as cryosurgical ablation, cryotherapy, or "cryo."

**CT scan (CAT scan)**: A 'computerized tomography' (CT) or 'computerized axial tomography' (CAT) scan uses a computer that takes data from several X-ray images of structures inside a human's or animal's body and converts them into pictures on a monitor.

**Cystitis**: Inflammation of the urinary bladder.

**Cytogenetic**: The branch of biology that deals with heredity and the cellular components such as chromosomes.

**D**

**Diabetes**: A metabolic disorder, sometimes marked by a persistent thirst, in which excessive amounts of glucose (sugar) is found within the bloodstream. Generally refers to one of the two types of diabetes mellitus, insulin-dependent and non-insulin-dependent.

**Dialysis**: A medical procedure in which metabolic waste products and toxic substances are removed from the blood using a machine. Dialysis is required for individuals with severe kidney failure.

**DNA**: Also known as deoxyribonucleic acid. DNA is the building block of the genes that encode for each of the proteins present in the body's cells. Each gene contains an ordered sequence of the four nucleotides and are comprised of matched pairs of nucleotides (A with T, C with G, etc.) and the two strands of DNA (A, adenine; C, cytosine; G, guanine; T, thymine).

**E**

**Echogenic**: The pattern of sound waves detected during an ultrasound examination. Kidney tumors can have increased or decreased echogenicity on ultrasound when compared to normal kidney. The main advantages of ultrasonography are that it is very safe and relatively inexpensive, but it often must be combined with other tests to yield a definitive diagnosis.

**Erythrocytosis**: An increase in red blood cell count numbers in the blood stream that can be seen in kindey cancer patients. It is thought to be due to increased production of a stimulatnt of red blood cell production, called erythropoietin.

**Erythropoietin**: A hormone that stimulates production of red blood cells and hemoglobin in the bone marrow. This hormone is overproduced by some kidney tumors leading to high red blood cell counts, the opposite of anemia.

**F**

**Familial**: Occurring in the members of a family: a familial disease.

**Flank**: The side of a human, also known as the retroperitoneum. This is where the kidney can be asccessed during open or laparoscopic surgery, or by bipopsy.

**G**

**Gene**: A segment of DNA that typically encodes a specific protein. Each gene contains an ordered sequence of the four nucleotides (A, C, G, and T).

**Genetic counseling**: The counseling of individuals with established or potential genetic problems. This specialty is concerned with inheritance patterns and risks to other related family members, such as siblings and children.

**Genetic mutation**: Change in the individual nucleotides of a gene that result in a change in the function or amount of that gene's protein product. Most nucleotide changes have no effect ("silent mutation"), but other mutations can have minor or major effects that can lead to disordered cell growth and cancer.

**Genome**: The total amount of genetic information in the chromosomes of an organism, including its genes and DNA sequences. The human genome is made up of about 35,000 genes.

**Glomeruli**: Glomeruli are knots of blood vessels in the kidney where the blood flows in, the urine is produced, and then the filtered blood flows out. Each knot projects into the end of a urine-secreting tubule near the capsule of the kidney.

**Glomerulonephritis**: A kidney disease affecting the small blood vessels of the glomeruli of the kidney, characterized by leakage of protein into the urine (albuminuria), fluid retention within the body(edema), and high blood pressure (hypertension).

**Glomerular filtration rate (GFR)**: A test to determine how well the kidneys are working. The estimate is based on the rate at which the kidneys filter the waste product creatinine from the bloodstream. According to the National Kidney Foundation, normal values range between 90 and

120 ml/min/1.73m². GFR values fall with age, so older people generally have lower values. Levels below 60 ml/min/1.73m² indicate mild to moderate chronic kidney disease and below 15 ml/min/1.73m² indicate kidney failure.

# H

**Hematocrit**: Blood test that measures the thickness of the blood, which is a reflection of its oxygen-carrying capacity. The hematocrit value is the ratio of the volume occupied by packed red blood cells to the volume of the whole blood.

**Hematuria**: The presence of blood in the urine.

**Hemoglobin**: The oxygen-carrying component in red blood cells that gives them their red color and serves to bring oxygen to the tissues.

**High blood pressure**: Elevation of the arterial blood pressure, also known as hypertension.

**Hypervascular**: Increased number of blood vessels supplying a tumor. Kidney cancer is typically hypervascular due to the high expression of the growth factor VEGF.

# I

**Immune system**: The body system in humans and other animals that protects the organism by distinguishing foreign tissue and neutralizing potentially pathogenic

organisms or substances. The immune system includes organs such as the skin and mucous membranes, which provide an external barrier to infection, cells involved in the immune response, such as lymphocytes, and cell products such as lymphokines.

**Immunogenicity**: The property of eliciting an immune response.

**Immunohistochemistry**: Microscopic localization of specific antigens in tissues by staining with antibodies labeled with fluorescent pigmented material.

**Immunosuppressive medication**: Drugs given to a transplant recipient to prevent his or her immune system from attacking the transplanted organ.

**Inherited**: To receive (a characteristic) from one's parents by genetic transmission.

**Intraoperative ultrasound (IOUS)**: Intraoperative ultrasound is a dynamic imaging modality that provides interactive and timely information during surgical procedures.

**Intravenous**: Within or through the blood; usually refers to medications or fluids given through an IV line.

# K

**Kidney**: Either of the two organs in the lumbar region that filter the blood, excreting the end-products of body metabolism in the form of urine, and regulating the concentrations of hydrogen, sodium, potassium, phosphate, and other ions in the extracellular fluid.

**Kidney failure:** Inability of the kidneys to excrete waste, which results in a person's inability to maintain a balance of fluid and electrolytes, such as sodium and potassium.

# L

**Laparoscopic:** Pertaining to laparoscopy, such as laparoscopic surgery. A fiber optic camera and instrument, passed through a small incision in the abdominal wall and equipped with instruments with which to examine the abdominal cavity or perform surgery. Some laparoscopic surgeries are also performed with a robotic surgical system, and termed "robot-assisted laparoscopic"or "robotic" surgeries.

**Laparoscopy:** Use of small instruments and telescopes (cameras that look inside the body) to access various compartments of the body. Carbon dioxide gas is pumped into the body through small channels in order to create space between the abdominal wall and the intraabdominal organs facilitating the operation.

**Lethal:** Capable of causing death.

# M

**Magnetic resonance imaging (MRI):** A patient is placed in a magnetic field and radiofrequency signals are transmitted and received by surrounding coils. A computer processes the information and constructs cross-sectional images which provide detailed information on soft tissues.

**Malignant:** The term literally means growing worse and resisting treatment. It is used as a synonym for cancerous and connotes a harmful condition that generally is life threatening.

**Malnutrition:** Lack of proper nutrition; inadequate or unbalanced nutrition.

**Medullary cell carcinoma:** An aggressive kidney cancer that occurs almost exclusively in patients with sickle cell trait or disease. Therefore, younger African Americans are most often affected.

**Metastasis:** Transmission of cancerous cells from an original site to one or more sites elsewhere in the body, usually by way of the blood vessels or lymphatics.

**Morcellate:** Because minimally-invasive, laparoscopic techniques use only small incisions, some surgeons have performed this technique to break larger specimens into smaller pieces so they can be removed without making a larger incision. This has not been done routinely for cancer specimens so that they can be examined as whole tumors by the pathologist after they have been removed.

**Multifocal**: Refers to having more than one tumor. Multifocal kidney cancer does not appear to be associated with worse prognosis, but can be a sign of an inherited kidney cancer.

**Mutations**: Changes in chromosomes or genes that cause proteins to function abnormally and begin a "cancerous process." Mutations can be caused by the effects of chemicals, radiation, or even ordinary heat on DNA.

# N

**Neoadjuvant therapy**: Treatment given as a first step to shrink a tumor before the main treatment, which is usually surgery, is given. Examples of neoadjuvant therapy include chemotherapy, radiation therapy, and hormone therapy. It is a type of induction therapy.

**Nephrectomy**: Surgical removal of a kidney.

**Nephrologist**: A physician subspecialized in managing nonsurgical kidney disease, who is board-certified in internal medicine and nephrology.

**Nomogram**: A predictive model that estimates the likelihood of a given outcome (such as recurrence of cancer or death due to cancer) based on specific characteristics of an individual patient and his or her cancer. Nomograms are intended to be user-friendly versions of complicated predictive models, and they are often available for doctors and patients in paper based formats or even online. www.cancernomograms.com is a website that allows simple input of clinical characteristics into kidney cancer nomograms that then allows the user to estimate risk of a given outcome (see Figure 20).

# O

**Oncogene**: An oncogene is a mutation that activates a cell and transforms it into a cancer. An activated oncogene is analogous to having the accelerator of a car stuck in the "on position," the cell then divides out of control, gathers other mutations, and becomes malignant.

**Oncologist**: A specialist in oncology, dealing with the diagnosis and medical treatment of cancer.

**Oncology**: The branch of medicine that deals with the diagnosis and treatment of cancer.

**Ophthalmologist**: A medical doctor specializing in the diagnosis and treatment of diseases of the eye.

# P

**Palpate**: To examine by feeling and pressing with the palms of the hands and the fingers.

**Papillary renal cell carcinoma**: The second most common subtype of kidney cancer, responsible for 10–15% of RCC. It is often multifocal with multiple lesions within one or both kidneys. Tends to display less aggressive clinical behavior.

**Paraneoplastic syndrome**: A disorder caused by the release of certain compounds by the kidney cancer cells.

**Parathormone**: A hormone synthesized and released into the bloodstream by the parathyroid glands; regulates phosphorus and calcium in the body and functions in neuromuscular excitation and blood clotting.

**Partial nephrectomy**: Removal of the portion of the kidney that contains the tumor, along with just enough healthy kidney to provide a safe margin.

**Percutaneous**: With regards to kidney cancer, refers to treatments performed by inserting a needle through the skin without further need for incisions.

**Peritoneum**: The serous membrane lining the walls of the abdominal and pelvic cavities and investing the contained viscera , the two layers enclosing a potential space, the peritoneal cavity.

**Placebo**: A sugar pill that is given in clinical trials in order to help determine whether the effect seen with the real medication is due to the treatment itself or due to other reasons (placebo effect).

**Proteases**: Enzymes that degrade protein molecules.

**Protein**: Proteins are fundamental components of all living cells and include many substances, such as enzymes, hormones, and antibodies, that are necessary for the proper functioning of an organism. They are found in foods such as meat, fish, eggs, milk, and legumes.

**Protocol**: The plan for a course of medical treatment or for a clinical trial.

# R

**Radiation therapy**: Treatment of disease by means of X-rays or radioactive substances.

**Radical nephrectomy**: The surgical removal of a kidney, usually performed in the treatment of cancer of the kidney.

**Radiofrequency ablation**: An energy-based technology that uses alternating current to heat tissue, thereby causing direct cell death and injury and destruction of the tumor's blood supply.

**Radiographic tests**: An examination performed to visualize parts of the body that are not visible with the naked eye. These tests use some form of energy to "see"a person's insides. Common types include plain X-ray, tomography (CT), magnetic resonance imaging (MRI), and ultrasound (US).

**Rejection**: The failure of a recipient's body to accept a transplanted tissue or organ as the result of immunological incompatability; immunological resistance to foreign tissue.

**Renal**: Relating to the kidney.

**Renal cell carcinoma (RCC)**: Cancer of the kidney.

**Renin**: A hormone of high specificity that is released by the kidney and acts to raise blood pressure by activating angiotensin.

**Resect**: To remove or excise tissue or part (or all) of an organ.

**Retroperitoneal**: The space between the peritoneum and the posterior abdominal wall that contains the kidneys, adrenal glands, pancreas, and part of the aorta and inferior vena cava.

**Risk–benefit ratio**: Counting the cost before making a decision, thinking of both the harms and benefits of acting and the changes that they will occur.

**Robot-assisted laparoscopic surgery**: Some laparoscopic surgeries are performed with a robotic surgical system, and termed "robot-assisted laparoscopic" or "robotic" surgeries. The surgeon is involved from the start to finish, performing the surgery with the assistance of the surgical robot.

**Robotic**: See robot-assisted laparoscopic surgery.

## S

**Satellite lesion**: Smaller tumors that grow near, but separate from the main renal cancer within the same kidney.

**Secrete**: To release a substance produced within cells out into the blood, urine, or other body fluid.

**Sequester**: To detach or separate abnormally a small portion from the whole.

**Serum creatinine**: The creatinine blood test measures the level of creatinine in the blood. This test is done to see how well your kidneys work.

**Sporadic**: Occurring at random or by chance, and not as a result of a genetically determined, or inherited, trait.

## T

**Thermal ablation**: Destruction of a tumor using heat or cold to disrupt the cancer cells and blood vessels.

**Transabdominal**: Across the abdominal wall or through the abdominal cavity.

**Transesophageal echocardiogram (TEE)**: A technique used to visualize the heart and major blood vessels. In this version of echocardioghraphy, the probe is placed inside the esophagus and for that reason is done when the person is asleep (under anesthesia).

**Transperitoneal**: Through the peritoneum, the smooth membrane that lines the abdominal cavity.

**Transplantation** : To transfer (an organ, tissue, etc.) from one part of the body to another or from one person or animal to another. Kidney transplantation from a living donor or a brain-dead accident victim can restore renal function to a patient without functioning kidneys.

**Tumor**: An abnormal growth of tissue, which can be benign or malignant. Similar to the term neoplasm, but should be distinguished from the term cancer, which implies at least some malignant potential.

**Tumor ablation**: Killing tumor cells directly using heat or cold or other type of energy. This is done laparoscopically or by percutaneous treatment.

**Tumor grade**: Tumor grade is a way of classifying tumors based on certain features of their cells. The grade of a tumor is directly linked to prognosis. Using a microscope, a pathologist studies the tumor tissue removed during a biopsy to check: 1) How much the cancer cells look like normal cells (The more the cancer cells look like normal cells, the lower the tumor grade tends to be.) 2) How many of the cancer cells are in the process of dividing (The fewer cancer cells that are in the process of dividing, the more likely it is that the tumor is slow-growing slowly and the lower the tumor grade tends to be.) Together, these two factors determine the tumor grade.

**Tumor suppressor gene**: A gene that codes for a protein that serves to regulate cell division and prevent cancer growth. When the gene is mutated so that the protein is either not made or cannot function, tumor growth is able to grow in an uncontrolled manner.

# U

**Ultrasound (US)**: An imaging modality that relies on sound waves that are transmitted through the skin, into the body, and detected by a transducer.

**Ureters**: The paired structures that carry urine from each kidney to the bladder.

**Urethra**: The canal through which urine is discharged from the bladder.

**Urine**: Liquid waste product filtered from the blood by the kidneys, stored in the bladder, and expelled from the body through the urethra by the act of urinating (voiding). About 96% of urine is water, with the remaining 4% being comprised of waste products.

**Urologist**: A physician who specializes in urology, including the clinical, surgical, and scientific aspects of the genitourinary tract in health and disease.

# V

**Vascular**: Pertaining to, composed of, or provided with vessels or ducts that convey fluids, as blood or lymph.

**Vascular endothelial growth factor (VEGF)**: A protein that is made within cells and released into the bloodstream. When cancer cells release VEGF, it stimulates the growth of new blood vessels, a process called angiogenesis. Although VEGF is just one of many factors that function in this way, it appears to play the major role in kidney cancer (and many other types of cancer).

**Vein**: Blood vessel that carries blood away from an organ, such as the kidney.

**Venogram**: An X-ray of the veins produced by venography.

**Viscosity**: The resistance of a substance to flow.

**von Hippel-Lindau (VHL) gene**: The von Hippel-Lindau tumor suppressor, also known as pVHL, is a protein that in humans is encoded by the VHL gene.

**von Hippel-Lindau syndrome (VHL)**: A genetic disease caused by mutation of a tumor suppressor gene that has been called the VHL gene. Mutation of this gene is the most common cause of familial kidney cancer and also occurs in the majority of noninherited clear cell RCC.

# W

**Wilms' tumor**: A malignant kidney tumor occurring in young children and composed of small spindle cells and other tissue.

**Note:** Page numbers followed by *f* and *t* indicate materials in figures and tables respectively.